Paul R

KU-678-870

Souls to Soles

A SELF-HELP EXPLORATION
OF REFLOXOLOGY

LOTUS LIGHT
SHANGRI-LA

This book is dedicated to my young daughter
Rachel
who has been a tremendous inspiration for bringing
this book to life. From a very early age she has
benefited from reflexology and is proud to
acknowledge the connection of her feet...
to the rest of her body.

To you, the reader, a dedication is made for taking
the time to explore reflexology. By doing so, you will
be learning to honor "a gift from the universe" that
lies within your own body.

Many people have knowingly contributed in their own
special ways to the evolution of this work. Their
support, guidance, wisdom and love, have given this
project special scope and direction. Included are my
mother, wife, family, friends and reflexology clients.

A special dedication is wished for several professional
colleagues who have each added significantly to this
project. To Dr. Flora Attias for her infinite wisdom and
supportive insights; to Op. Dr. M. F. Abut for having
introduced me to the true nature of healing; to Bill
Flocco for his superlative training and ethical
approaches to reflexology; to Jean Lanford for her
spiritual guidance and for always being available as
a constructive critic; and to Christine Issel for helping
me to focus on techniques for the young, and for
supporting this work with her words of introduction and
expansive approach to reflexology.

I am eternally grateful to all of you.

Paul Rudé

April 1995

Paul Rudé has written *Souls to Soles* for enthusiasts of all ages, for both givers and receivers of reflexology. Paul has made reflexology simple, but not simplistic. In his own unique style he has captured the essence of reflexology in a concise way while giving it the reverence and respect it so richly deserves. On a practical level he makes learning easy while upholding the proper ethics and attitudes necessary for effective touch work. This is the heart of *Souls to Soles*.

Paul balances the sensitive side of the work with his well developed sense of humor. A unique part of the book are Paul's original illustrations and the homework assignments. Believe it or not, you won't want to skip over these pages! Everyone will find the coloring assignments great fun. They can be used as a teaching tool for students of reflexology, to reinforce and test your own understanding, and a great way to share reflexology with young ones. Every reader will enjoy the word searches, crossword puzzles and "colorful" exercises.

On a more serious note, we know that from cradle to grave, reflexology is beneficial and has been found to be a soothing non-invasive technique. Yet, an often overlooked area of emphasis is the use of reflexology with children. Since children are our future, they especially deserve to receive the benefits of reflexology. Caring for infants, however, poses special challenges since they are not able to communicate about their health stresses. Paul's contribution of Light Touch Reflex Action (LTRA) makes this book very valuable in this regard.

Care givers who have been at their wits' end because of a cranky or ill child will readily appreciate the guidelines set forth for working with the young. The feet can communicate to us what infants or children are unable to verbalize. Reflexology is a way of nurturing them in an immediate way. It allows the care giver to express concern, to do something helpful in a concrete way, and to ease the discomforts, all at the same time. We feel better and so do they! At anytime, at any age, reflexology is a way of sharing. With my own children over the years, I found that doing reflexology with them was a time of sharing. Regardless of their age, they would let me know what was going on in their lives and what their concerns were without my prying. This was particularly important in the teen years. In both directions, between giver and receiver, reflexology truly works from **soul** to **sole**.

There's always something new to learn, and every author has gems of wisdom to impart. Paul has managed to present a book which has elements for everyone, at all interest levels - from students of reflexology to professional reflexologists, from grand-parents

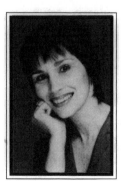

and parents to the children. As reflexology emerges into its own profession, *Souls to Soles* is a welcome addition to its expanding library.

Christine Issel

Author - Reflexology: Art, Science & History
Founder of local, state, national and international reflexology organizations.

THE BASICS

• What you need to know •

THE REFERENCES
• What you should explore •

Congratulations for having taken a step towards paying more attention to your feet! By doing so, you will be giving your body a most natural and powerful stimulus for promoting and maintaining well being. Reflexology is rapidly becoming accepted worldwide as a unique **complementary** health modality. It's a profession unto itself, and a most effective tool for self-help health care. Medical care and health care are **separate issues**. Everyone has a right to search for natural self-help therapies which support **well being**. The main concept of reflexology is its ability to balance the body and mind in a safe and effective manner regardless of age and health status.

Just as roots are important to plants, feet are important to human beings. They're a **wonder of nature** but receive so very little attention.

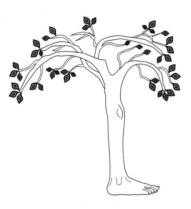

This book is an introduction to working with the feet, and it's meant to be a companion guide... something to have handy, to help you deal with the stresses and strains of everyday life. We all know only too well that the negative effects of stress are taking their toll in an unprecedented way. Even the established medical profession recognizes the importance of stress reduction, attributing up to 80 percent of today's ailments to stress-related factors.

Stress has become an ugly word in our vocabulary, conjuring up all kinds of negative emotions. It's used at the drop of a pin to explain so many situations. Try listening around you for a few days and note the many ways the word is used. Stress has certainly taken its toll! For some it's become monumental... to the point of daily **exhaustion**!

A certain amount of stress will always be present in our lives. Think of it as a stimulus (both negative and positive). Without a certain amount of stress in the body we wouldn't be living beings. Accumulated negative stress is what plays havoc with the mind and body. To understand this concept just hold on to an ugly or negative thought for a moment. Notice how

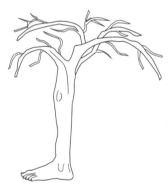

your body tenses up? Now think of this tension as layers of your life that accumulate as blockages of energy in your feet. That's what this book is about, and how you can **help** your **life**... **through your feet**.

This book also extends reflexing to children. Adults have the ability to search for meaningful stress reducers but children don't. They're largely dependent on adults to ease their stresses. This exploration of reflexology will help you **reach out** to them... in a **new** and **meaningful way** that focuses on specific touch techniques to the feet.

A... **B**... **C**... **D**... it's really that simple!

This book is organized on **2 levels** as you saw in the table of contents. The Basics and The References.

If reflexology is a **new experience** for you, it's essential that you progress through "The Basics", **step-by-step**. By doing so, you'll be learning in a logical order.

Sections A & B are crucial for you to understand:

• how reflexes relate to body parts,

• what kind of touch to use,

• what a tender reflex is,

• what the cautions are.

Section C introduces the foot reflex guides to help you use your touch effectively.

Section D is for infant and child reflexology, and is based on your understanding the preceding sections.

Section W expands on the foot reflex guide concept of Section C with extra details about reflexes. Learning is reinforced in a fun way with charts that you can color code, and blank charts for your own use.

Section X further reinforces reflex concepts with crossword puzzles and word search games.

Section Y is where you'll find reference information.

Section Z has associations/book lists and the index.

Many of the pages in this book have been organized as **paired** pages focusing on :

• a specific topic or concept,

• a matching of body areas to foot reflex guides.

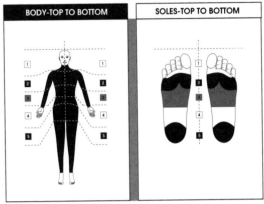

BODY-TOP TO BOTTOM	SOLES-TOP TO BOTTOM

Left/Right pages are organized with matching numbers to find the body-foot relationship.
Body number boxes are either white, gray or black to match the reflex area shading.

SYMBOLS USED IN THE BOOK

Key points to remember well

Indicates reflexing an area on the side of the foot

Specifies glands or structures involved in immune functions

NOTE ON IMMUNITY: Immune functions of the body are complex processes. Chemical and electrical communication within the body **supports** immunity by **balancing** body **energy**, thereby promoting resistance to disease. This book focuses on immune functions in a broad manner by including the main reflexes that support these chemical/electrical functions. They are labeled for reflexing in Sections **C** & **W**.

READ ME FIRST

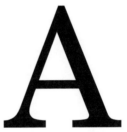

A

**READ ME
FIRST**

Greetings! My name is Little Foot. I'll be your helper as we explore the wonderful world of reflexology.

The short time it takes to read the essentials of this book should prove to be an **investment** for your **well being**. You'll be learning a skill which can help you dramatically with the stresses of everyday life.

Once you've understood the basics about footcare and "reflexing" you'll be able to refer to the drawings at any time, and use your touch effectively!

Read on with a smile!

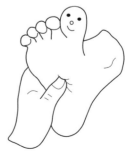

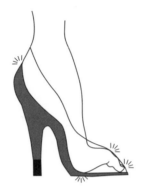

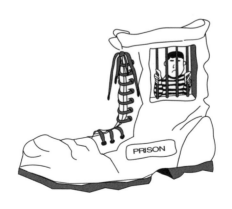

PRISON

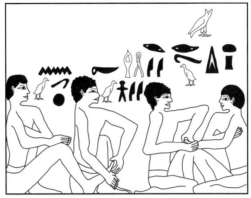

Pictogram from the Egyptian tomb of Ankhmahor
(circa 2500 B.C.)

Our feet are too often the most **neglected** parts of our bodies! This is unfortunate since they literally "carry us through life". Stimulating the feet is a **natural** touch therapy which has been used for thousands of years. It's been a part of the culture of ancient civilizations such as Egypt, China and India. In more recent times, the relationship between the body and the feet has been well mapped out and refined within the unique modality known today as **reflexology**.

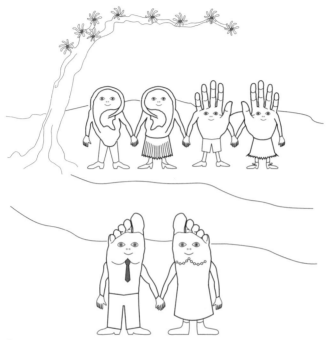

Caring for the feet has no specific history or roots. It could very well be that we started touching our feet for therapeutic reasons ever since our days as cave people. Throughout history, touching the feet has had special meaning, bringing to mind scenes of compassion and caring touch for the weak or wounded, and for those of special **soul**.

The hands and ears also have a rich history which should be noted even though this book focuses on the feet. Reflexology is broadly defined as a touch modality that is applied to complete localized maps that resemble **a shape of the body**. We'll be exploring the foot maps, but it just so happens that the hands and ears also have their own full maps that resemble a shape of the body.

Reflex areas are like **push buttons** that send messages to the rest of the body. The **sum total** of these reflex areas is like a telephone touch pad that looks a lot like your body. These "buttons" are often confused with acupressure or acupuncture points. Reflexology is **a system of its very own**. There are lots of specific points on the body used for these other therapies, but they're learned with great precision in order to be effective. Reflexology is more **forgiving** and **easy** to learn for several reason:

• the reflex areas are quite **broad**, and after getting the basic idea about the body-foot relationship, you'll be able to **navigate** your body and then navigate the foot to use your touch,

• the parts of the body under stress, pain or imbalance show up as **tender spots** in the reflex areas,

• the maps are easy to follow since they represent a logical **mirrored image** of the body. If you have a general idea about body parts, and most people do, then you can learn about reflexing. Whether the body is small (infant/child), medium (teenage), or large (adult), the reflexes relate to the body, not just to the reflexology maps or charts, of which there are so many.

Ultimately, your **own body** will be your guide for finding the effective place to reflex, and once you get comfortable with reflexing the feet, you might even be led to experiment with your hands and outer ears!

You feel good when you're relaxed!

Good relaxation can have a profound effect on our **ability to cope** with the negative stresses of life, and it just so happens that stresses accumulate in the reflex areas as blockages of energy. When the reflex areas are normalized the rest of your body benefits! It's still something of a mystery as to how reflex areas are connected to the rest of the body, and how they get "blocked up". There are several theories as to how all of this works. The most accepted one proposes that the rich supply of nerve endings (7,000+) in the feet send messages all over the body through the nervous system - (see B- 28 & 29).

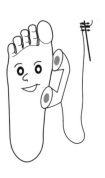

An analogy can be made with a telephone system: when you dial a number, you get a certain person on the other end of the telephone. The reflex areas work to communicate as well. But when they call up a part of the body, it's to say... **RELAX!**

This relaxation is at the cellular level. Cells make up tissues, and tissues make up body organs and structures. So when the body has a chance to relax, the cells themselves are benefiting and doing their jobs better. They're getting more energy from blood nutrients, more oxygen and a more normal delivery of electrical impulses. All of this helps to **normalize** body functions and reduce or eliminate pains, ultimately improving vitality.

An automobile works properly when it's tuned up. Likewise, an orchestra sounds good only when all the instruments are in tune. The body's the same. Health is like a **symphony**! When all the body parts are tuned and relaxed, there's more energy and more resistance to ailments and diseases.

Does the body talk to itself, grumble or sing? Of course, you can get a headache when the stomach is upset. Pain anyplace in the body can leave you totally off-center! The body works **together** as one, and even your thought patterns have their effects on the body.

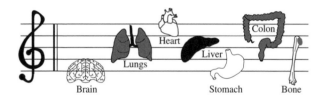

Reflexology is unique as a self-help process. It's easy to learn, and wonderful to **share** with loved ones. It can be used for acute problems or for relief of stresses from chronic situations. You can use it preventively to optimize your chances for health, or to help feel better when your health fails you. There are many ailments and diseases, but there's only one harmony of health. Give yourself a better chance to function with more **body harmony**. Happy feet can lead the way to where there's absence of pain on the physical level, the spirit and emotions are light and positive and mental attitudes are sharp and focused. In essence, that's what health and harmony is all about.

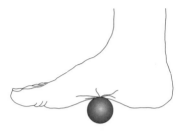

Rolling on a ball
(sitting... not standing)

In addition, there are many "reflex tools" available commercially for stimulating the feet such as foot rollers, electric massagers, pads to tread on. Refer to Section **Y** pages 8-11 for information on reflex tools and how to use them effectively.

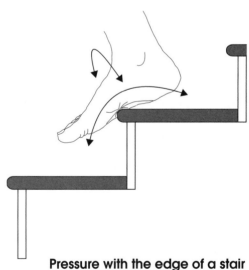

Pressure with the edge of a stair
(work on a low tread, and hold on to something solid for safety)

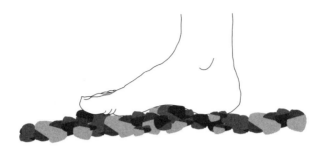

Walking on smooth stones
(...also sand, and wet grass)

Ever wonder why it feels so good to walk along the beach? Coming into contact with the ground is beneficial because electromagnetic forces from the earth travel into your body through your feet! Natural reflex stimulus through the feet is truly a wonder of nature. Animals benefit all the time since they don't wear shoes.

Before getting into the touch work, just be aware that there are other ways to work your feet besides using your thumb or finger pressure. Use your imagination... but use **common sense** at all times!

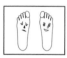

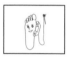

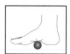

This page is meant to help you focus on some of the key points in Section A.
How many useful concepts or words come to mind?

B

**GETTING
STARTED**

General Overview

Now let's get down to business!
On the next page the body is divided into
three groups of body parts to introduce the
first **general rules of thumb** about reflexes:

1. - reflexes relating to the main part of the
body *(torso)* and the head are found mainly
on the **soles** of the feet,

2. - reflexes relating to the sides of the body
are found mainly on the **outside** of the feet,

3. - reflexes relating to the centerline of the
body are found mainly on the **inside**
edges of the feet.

Match the body **numbers**
to the foot numbers!

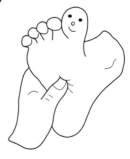

The 3 Main Body Divisions

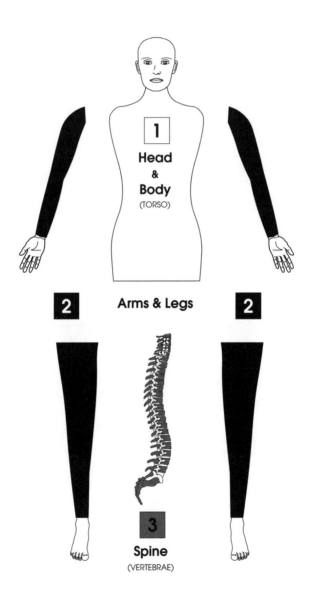

1

Head
&
Body
(TORSO)

2 Arms & Legs **2**

3

Spine
(VERTEBRAE)

GENERAL DIVISIONS - FOOT REFLEX AREAS

The 3 Main Reflex Divisions

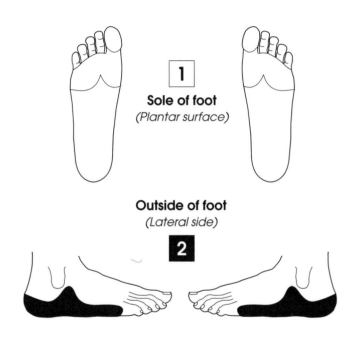

1

Sole of foot
(Plantar surface)

Outside of foot
(Lateral side)

2

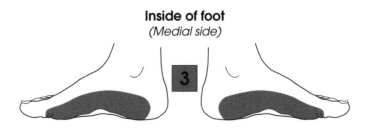

Inside of foot
(Medial side)

3

Match a body part listed in the boxed area below to a view of the feet that corresponds. Are the reflexes to be found on the sole or sides of the feet? For now, don't worry about matching left and right sides of the body and feet, that's for latter. You can color in the LETTERS of the headings with the same color as the matching feet.

✎ Use 3 colors for matching - 1 color for each **heading** and **the pair** of feet that corresponds.

1 - HEAD/BODY (TORSO)

2 - SPINE (VERTEBRAE)

3 - ARMS/LEGS

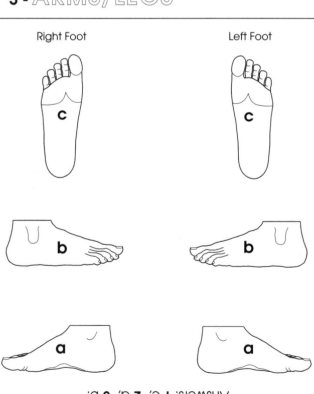

Right Foot   Left Foot

Answers: 1-c, 2-a, 3-b.

Top to Bottom

Next we'll look at everything from **top** to **bottom**.

The toes (top of the foot) correspond to the top of the body (head). Working our way down the foot and body, we'll see that there are **five** easily recognized **division areas** for the correspondences.

Again **match the body** numbers **to the foot** numbers.

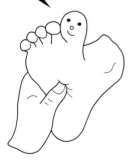

The 5 Main Division Areas

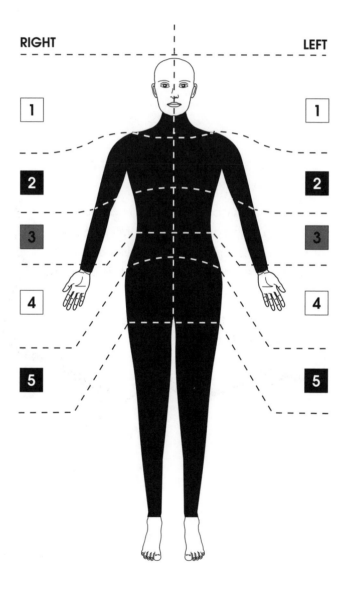

The 5 Main Reflex Divisions

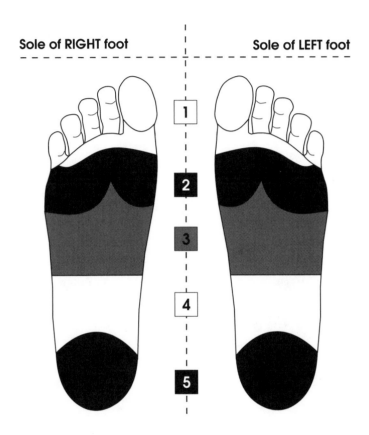

Sole of RIGHT foot | Sole of LEFT foot

MAIN DIVISION AREAS

1- Head and Neck
2- Chest and Shoulders
3- Upper Abdomen
4- Lower Abdomen
5- Pelvic Area

In the boxed area below you'll find 5 body labels. Use what you've learned about the 5 **main division areas** to match each label (1-5) to the division area of the foot where the reflex might be (a-e).

Again, don't worry about left and right correspondences yet, and have fun coloring if you wish.

✎ Use 5 colors, one for each label and the division area it matches on **each** foot. Both feet should have the same color for each division, like a rainbow.

---

1 - HEAD/NECK   **4 -** CHEST

2 - HIP   **5 -** STOMACH

3 - COLON

Sole of Right Foot

Sole of Left Foot

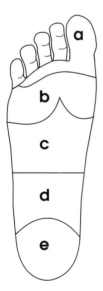

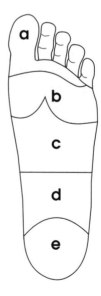

Answers: 1-a, 2-e, 3-d, 4-b, 5-c.

Right & Left

Now let's see how the right foot works the right side of the body, and the left foot, the left side of the body!

We'll just look at two examples for now:

1. - the **lungs** and,

2. - the **colon** (large intestine).

Once you get this concept, you'll be on your way to understanding how each foot may be used for **different** purposes.

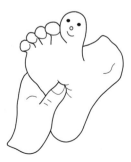

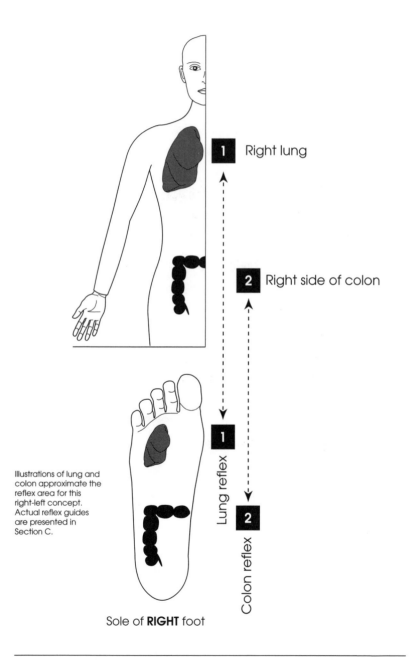

1 Right lung

2 Right side of colon

1 Lung reflex

2 Colon reflex

Illustrations of lung and colon approximate the reflex area for this right-left concept. Actual reflex guides are presented in Section C.

Sole of **RIGHT** foot

LEFT SIDE

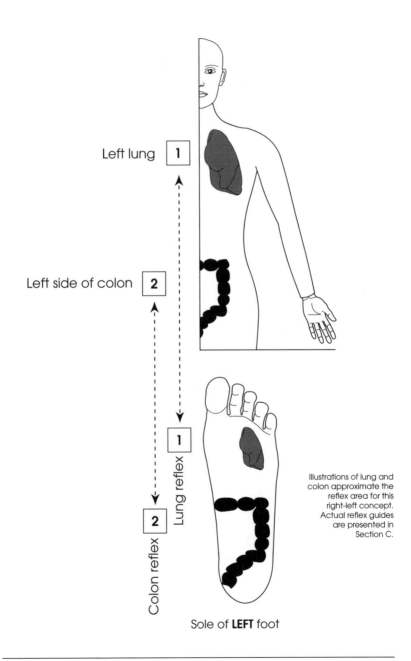

Left lung 1

Left side of colon 2

1 Lung reflex

2 Colon reflex

Illustrations of lung and colon approximate the reflex area for this right-left concept. Actual reflex guides are presented in Section C.

Sole of **LEFT** foot

Now let's put a few things together and see how we're doing! We should be able to match a body label to the correct left or right foot, and a general reflex area.

✎ Use 6 colors to match one heading to one letter on a foot. Code abbreviation: L. =Left - R. =Right

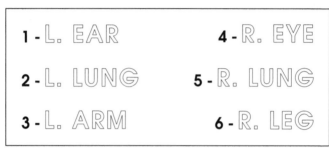

1 - L. EAR   4 - R. EYE

2 - L. LUNG   5 - R. LUNG

3 - L. ARM   6 - R. LEG

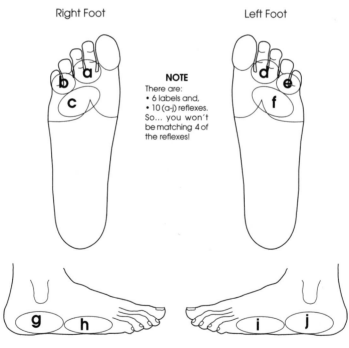

Right Foot   Left Foot

NOTE
There are:
• 6 labels and,
• 10 (a-j) reflexes.
So... you won't be matching 4 of the reflexes!

Answers: 1-e, 2-f, 3-i, 4-a, 5-c, 6-g.

NAVIGATING

By now you should have a pretty good idea about how the body relates to the feet... but we're going to make it even **easier** now!

On the next two pages you'll see how getting to the correct reflex area of the foot is a lot like how boats and planes get around the world... **by navigating.**

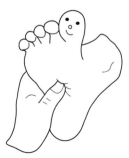

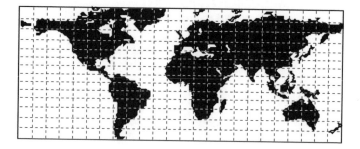

Finding the area on the foot that matches an area of the body is so easy that you may do it with your eyes closed. We'll call it **navigating**. Boats or planes get around without 'seeing'. They can navigate in the dark or in fog because the world has an artificial grid-like system known as longitude and latitude lines.

A similar type grid system may be used for reflexing. Actually, the foot was divided up like this thanks to Dr. W. Fitzgerald, and Dr. J. Riley in the early 1900's. A lot of what is presently considered reflexology is attributed to their work which was named **zone** therapy or zonery and in many parts of the world reflexology is referred to using this zone concept. Eunice Ingham added to their work to develop the mirrored image concept showing a shape of the body on the feet.

Latitude lines run east to west on the world map, and on the body they go **across** the body to outline the main division areas (1-5) which you saw on B-9. (not shown here... but you should be able to imagine them).

Longitude lines run north to south on the world map, and on the body they go from the head **down** into the fingers, and from the head **down** into the toes.

BODY ZONES

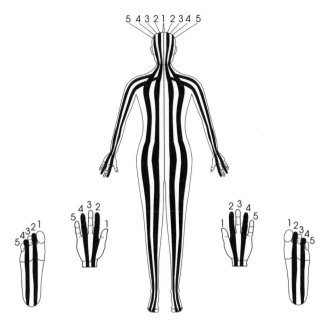

Dr. Fitzgerald discovered that an imbalance in the body could be **traced** along its zone to a reflex in the same zone of the foot or hand. This concept is great for navigating since it divides the body into five **imaginary zones** relating to each foot and hand.

Look at your body in a mirror now and trace five imaginary zones on each side of the **centerline** of your body. The zones go right through your body as well. Zone 1 in the center of the chest is also zone 1 in the center of the back. Now focus on a part of your body that carries stress or discomfort. If it's on the side of the body, that's zone 5! If it's in the middle of the back, that's zone 1. If it's in the chest area you have a choice of zones. Using zones is valuable as another **guide** for matching the body to the corresponding reflex area that you want to work with.

Now match reflexes to your **own body**! Navigate your body to find areas that carry stress or tension on a regular basis. Mark the correct foot and area to reflex. Provide labels or mark reflexes as you wish.

YOUR RIGHT FOOT   **YOUR LEFT FOOT**

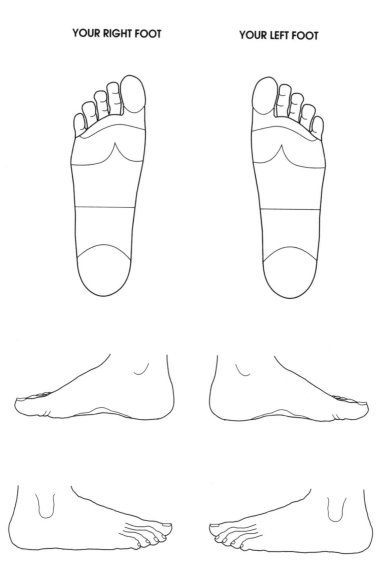

Pressure & Action

Now we'll learn how to use our touch. We want to be **effective** with our touch so we'll be learning a mainstream technique known as **thumbwalking**.

We don't want to get our thumb all stressed out, so we'll learn how to use the right combination of **force**, **pressure** and **support**. We're going to meet tender spots on the foot, but don't be put off, everybody has them, we're going to work with them!

Start practicing with the next few pages. You might want to try the thumbwalk on the palm of a **hand** before going to a foot... that way you can practice anywhere without taking off a shoe or sock!

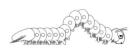

The **normal** pressure to use for reflexing is about the pressure you would use to crush a ripe grape. It's helpful to actually try this out. Imagining the pressure while you're reading this is one thing. It's great to actually feel your thumb pushing into the grape. So when you get a chance grab a few to experiment with!

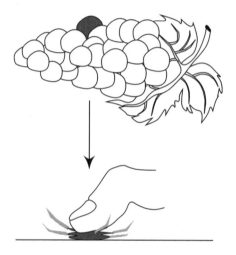

This is a general rule, however, and pressure should be **adjusted** for the person being reflexed. For children, the elderly, the very sick or very weak, the pressure will be **lighter** in most cases. The same is true for very sensitive individuals. If you aren't sure about your touch, the best guide is to start off lightly, and gradually apply more pressure. You may always go deeper with your touch as you work the area. If you go too deep right away, you might stress up your body in response to the strong stimulus. If you choose to work on others, be sensitive to their comfort level and **watch** their **responses** as you reflex for them.

Anybody may have tender spots on their feet. Even very healthy people can have tender spots. Normal daily stress may leave the feet feeling tender to the touch! The object of reflexing is to work with the tendernesses by applying **appropriate** pressure.

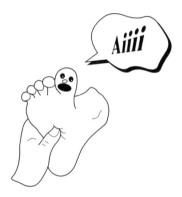

For those of you new to reflexing, it's real common to wonder what the tender spots are! When you start applying pressure to a foot (or a hand or ear), it's common to hear "**What's That For... ?!#**". Just remember that it's not always the reflex! There may be several reasons why there are tender spots, including:

- Problems with the bones or old injuries ,
- A wound, bruise or sprain in the area,
- Problems with a muscle or tendon ,

AND

- A **blockage** of **energy** between the **reflex** and the corresponding area of the body.

Now that we know about pressure and what to expect with tender spots, let's see how to get the thumb into **action**. Our little friend here is a great example.

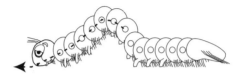

A caterpillar moves itself forward on a surface with a gliding, **wavelike** action. You're going to be using the same kind of action when you reflex. The caterpillar uses **leverage** from its **body** to push forward. You too can use a bit of leverage from your body. It comes from your shoulder area. You just let a little bit of force travel down your arm, right into the first joint of your thumb. It's **not a pushing action** from the shoulder, it's just being aware that your shoulder should be up there **supporting** the action on the foot.

This gentle body force helps the thumb's first joint move forward with the wavelike action on the skin surface. If you don't use this trick, your thumb will get tired too quickly. It'll be doing all the work on its own, and it doesn't need to! When you've had a bit of practice you might even develop a kind of **rhythm** with the wavelike action.

You don't want to tire out one thumb too much at a time. Alternate between using each hand and thumb. You may also use other fingers, especially the index and middle fingers, but in general the thumb will be able to apply the most effective wavelike pressure.

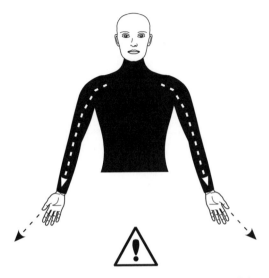

Don't jab at the foot with your thumb!

Reflexing is a combination of smooth force and pressure that starts in the shoulder area and ends up as **micro-movements** of the thumb on the surface of the foot.

Keep the caterpillar concept in your mind...
...and in your thumb!

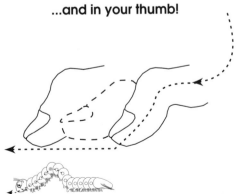

MICRO - MOVEMENTS

This is not like massage which uses broader actions of the hands. Reflexing is **micro-movements**! It's detailed work that's "pushing the buttons". Remember the telephone keyboard analogy!

The skin of your thumb or finger keeps in **contact**, pushing into the skin from the first joint. Move forward a little at a time (1/4"-1/2"). Use just the right amount of pressure to be effective but not cause undue discomfort on any tender spots. Push into the skin, slide forward and repeat the pressure as you go along.

You might experiment using talcum powder, lotion, cream or oil on the foot to help you move smoothly, but it isn't required. You want to reflex, not massage or slip all over the place, especially with the toes. Nevertheless, everyone has different likes and dislikes. So **experimentation** is in order here. Sometimes just the scent of baby powder or an aromatic oil may provide a special atmosphere for the touch work.

Remember that you may practice this reflex action on the palm of your hand before taking the shoes and socks off.

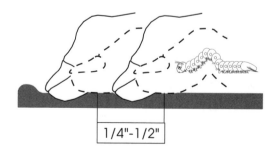

1/4"-1/2"

Let's put it all together now! One hand holds the foot to control its position while you reflex. The other hand does the reflexing. Note that the fingers of the reflexing hand are **supporting** the work of the thumb. Your fingers **always** backup or support the thumbwork, and should provide a good grip on any part of the foot while you reflex. For the toes, only a couple of fingers have room to back up the thumb, but when you reflex any other part of the foot, the fingers should be helping out to provide support for the reflex action on the foot (the same rules apply for reflexing on the hands).

The **combination** of force, pressure and support shown below is really the key for **effective micro-movements**.

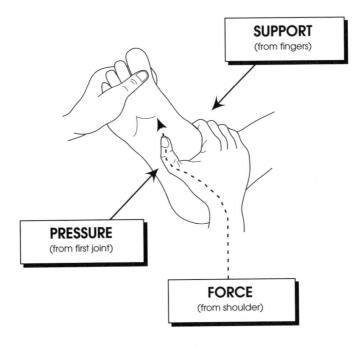

Reflexing another person's right foot
with your right hand.

Any time the body is worked with for therapeutic value certain cautions should be upheld. For reflexing they're minimal, but should be well noted:

•   The length of your nails might be a problem. The best reflexing is done with little or no nail to get in the way. You may get around this problem by adjusting the **angle of your thumb** to the reflex area. After a while it will become second nature to keep this angle just right, and not dig into the skin.
•   Using a '**tool**' instead of your touch is a real no-no when working on someone else unless you have a lot of experience with reflexology. A 'tool' is anything you might think of using on the foot to apply pressure as a substitute for your own touch. For more information on reflex tools, refer to that heading in Section **Y**.

Don't reflex over broken skin,

bruises

large varicose veins

wounds

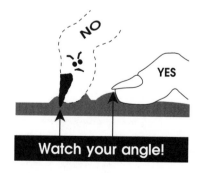

Watch your angle!

ONLY MEDICAL PROFESSIONALS ARE LICENSED TO
DIAGNOSE

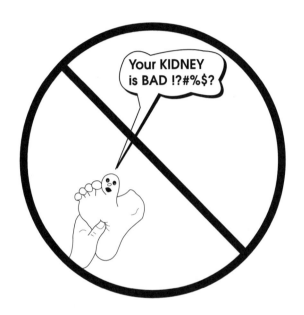

REMEMBER THAT THERE MAY BE SEVERAL REASONS WHY
A REFLEX AREA IS TENDER TO THE TOUCH.

SO DON'T MAKE AUTOMATIC ASSUMPTIONS ABOUT
"THE REFLEX " AND SOMETHING IN THE BODY!

THE OBJECT OF REFLEXING IS TO WORK WITH THE
TENDERNESS UNTIL IT EASES OR
THE STRESS IN THE BODY LESSENS.

**YOUR POSITIVE ATTITUDE TOWARDS TOUCHING
IS AS IMPORTANT AS THE TOUCH ITSELF**

Understanding how reflexology works is difficult to grasp because we're confronted by a new reality which our minds are not conditioned to accept. Do we really understand how a tulip seed knows how to grow into a tulip instead of crabgrass. Ultimately it's a mystery of the universe.

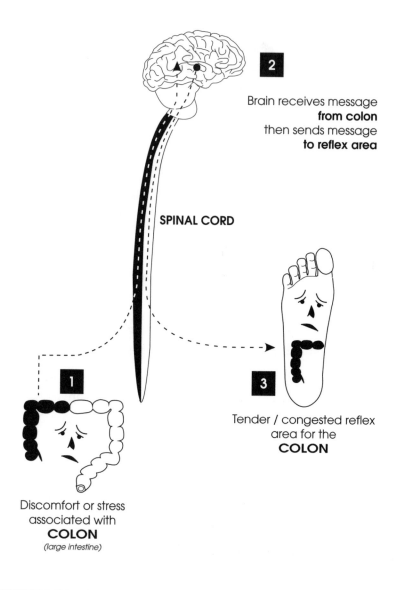

2

Brain receives message **from colon** then sends message **to reflex area**

SPINAL CORD

1

Discomfort or stress associated with **COLON** *(large intestine)*

3

Tender / congested reflex area for the **COLON**

THE REFLEX ACTION

We do know that a living organism functions because of universal energy which it uses for its own ends. Reflexology functions to improve or restore that process when things have gone wrong. The illustrations on these pages present one of the mainstream reflexology theories about this energy relationship, using the colon as a reflex example.

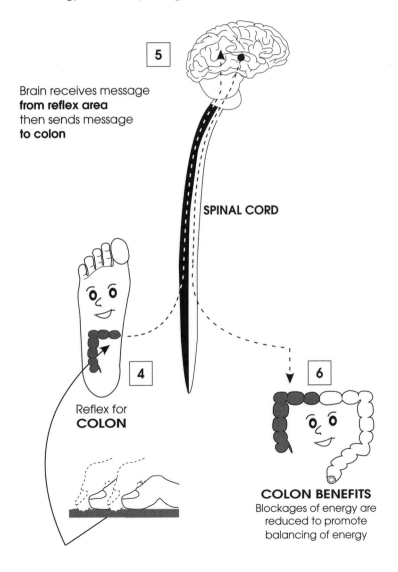

5

Brain receives message
from reflex area
then sends message
to colon

SPINAL CORD

4

Reflex for
COLON

6

COLON BENEFITS
Blockages of energy are
reduced to promote
balancing of energy

1. Reflexing has the ability to reduce or eliminate pain, and balance body energy. It also has the potential to stimulate the immune system, enabling the **"natural pharmacy"** of the body to function more effectively. Ultimately, the body and mind are helped to cope better with the negative effects of stress.

2. Reflexing may promote **toxin** release, especially when the feet are worked deeply or for more than 20 minutes. In this case, it's to your advantage to drink some extra water to help flush toxins from the body in a natural way.

3. Reflexing may be done at **any time** of the day or night: for a few minutes, concentrating on a certain reflex area, or a longer, more complete session as time allows you. Working **both feet completely** has wonderful revitalizing effects.

4. If there are tender spots on the foot, remember: DON'T DIAGNOSE. There may be **many reasons** why a reflex area is tender.

5. A tender reflex area means that extra attention should be given to that spot on the foot. Continue reflexing until the stress in the body starts to relax. When the problem in the body gets better, the **reflex** area will be **less tender**.

6. Each age group has the ability to derive appropriate benefits from reflexing. Remember to **adjust** your **touch** for the situation, level of stress and age. Start off lightly and gradually apply pressure.

7. If you choose to **help others**, it's always proper to ask permission, and to make them comfortable while you're working. If you are not an experienced reflexologist, using "tools" on others is not recommended.

8. Body cream, lotion, oil or talcum may be used on the feet if you wish, but is **not necessary**. Be careful not to hurt the foot with your nails.

9. When you get some practice reflexing, you'll probably note that tender areas feel **different** from the surrounding tissues. You might be able to **anticipate** tender spots! Managing any pain associated with reflex areas may be greatly assisted by breathing in deeply and exhaling slowly as the tenderness is reflexed.

10. Each person will react **differently** to reflexing. There may be shifts in body energy during and after reflexing. Sometimes the effect is energizing, and other times it's relaxing. Just as each personality is different, so is each person's reaction to a reflexing experience.

11. Use your **own body** as a guide to the reflex locations. Use the general division area and zone concepts to find the **broader area** of the foot to reflex.

12. Reflexology is not massage. **It's a system of its own.** It has the ability to reduce stresses by normalizing:

- blood circulation,
- energy flow to all parts of the body,
- immune functions,
- the spirit and emotions.

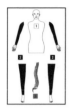

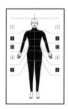

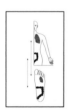

   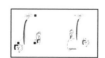

This page is meant to help you focus on some of the key points in Section B.
How many useful concepts or words come to mind?

C

FOOT
REFLEX GUIDES

FOOT REFLEX GUIDES

Maps... maps... maps... ! That's what usually comes to mind at first concerning reflexology. So let's have a look, but first we need to put a few things in perspective about maps.

One of the main focuses of this book is to help you navigate on your own instead of burying yourself in maps, but still we need them. The **mirrored** image concept helps us understand quickly. When you look at the images on the next page you can clearly see the way the feet correspond to the body. Nevertheless, the chart doesn't mean that the picture area on the foot is **directly** connected to the body parts. Nobody really knows for sure how the connection is made. There are only theories. The mirrored image concept just makes it easier to understand that **there is a connection**.

There are lots of published reflexology maps and charts. They're all somewhat different and this can be quite confusing! Why isn't there just one? First, people are different. Each person has their own size, shape and anatomy. Each of us is "wired" up differently as well. The nerve pathways connecting everything together can be different from one person to another. Remember the telephone analogy and that the feet have thousands of nerve ending. Well the reflex maps take all of this into account. That's why each map you see can be quite different. By the time you get comfortable with the contents of this book you'll be able to draw your own map in Section **W**.

MIRRORED IMAGES

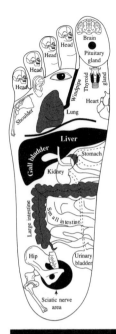

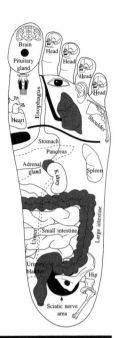

THERE IS NO PERFECT MAP THAT FITS EVERYBODY

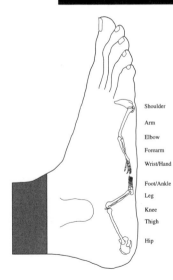

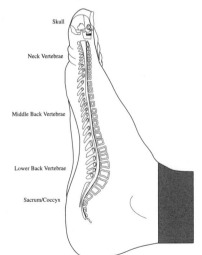

Now that you've looked at the 'mirrored image' let's put it aside and develop the reflex guides that make up the rest of this section.

In Section **B** you learned about navigating the body and the feet; how to search out those tender spots and relate them to the body. You might already have done this without the help of the maps. Nevertheless, maps are really useful and we'll get into the details after noting a few important considerations:

• You won't find all parts of the body on these maps. For the purposes of this book, only **major body parts** are referred to. Nevertheless, everything in the body is on the feet. It might not be on a map, but remember that the map isn't **your body**. In addition, it might not even be in your body! Surgery or birth defects can account for this. Nevertheless the reflex on the feet will correspond to that **area** of the body, but not the body part if you don't have it. So remember that the maps are only guides... and that's exactly what we're going to call them.

• You'll note that the maps for the right sole and left sole are different. The reason is simple! The body looks symmetrical outside, but **inside** the body, things are very different. When you study the body drawings you'll see this, and how each foot reflects this.

• Sometimes there's more than one area of the foot to reflex for an area of the body. So if you see a body part referred to more than once, it means that you should reflex any part of the foot that has a guide for that area.

- It's always important to reflex a **broad area** once you've found the general spot to use your touch on. When there's stress in a specific part of the body, it might be affecting a broader area in the body. A good example is for the spine. If there's stress in a particular vertebra, the bones, tissues and nerves below and above the affected vertebra might be under stress as well. The ability to relax a broad area of the body is one reason reflexing can be so powerful.

The **reflex guides** that start on the next page **match** body areas or parts to the reflexes. Use the **numbers** to find where to work with your touch. The rest of this section is organized as follows:

• **C 6-17** presents reflexes for the head and for the main parts of the body (torso).

• **C 18-25** presents reflexes for the rest of the body parts, and introduces the urinary and reproductive systems.

• **C 26 & 27** presents a summary view of reflex guides.

NOTE ON IMMUNE FUNCTIONS Immunity is largely a function of communication in the body. There are glands that secrete hormones into the blood stream to be carried to distant parts of the body. Electrical impulses must also reach their destinations all over the body. Many parts of the body are involved! Remember the analogy to the orchestra on A-9?

In this section and section **W - ᗕ** is the **symbol** used to label **major** body parts that either have a gland or a structure that may **support** immunity directly, or that supports it indirectly by balancing body energy.

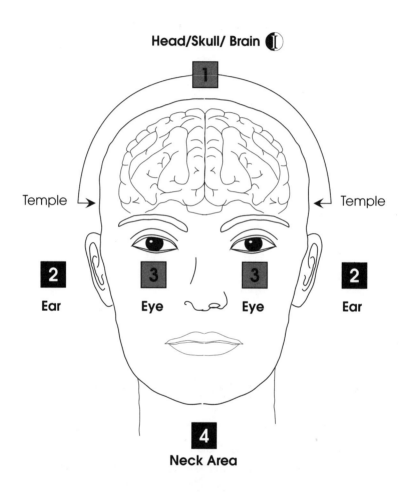

Head/Skull/ Brain

1

Temple → ← **Temple**

2 **3** **3** **2**
Ear **Eye** **Eye** **Ear**

4
Neck Area

On this first drawing of a body area, the eyes and ears are shown with a number for each side of the body.
For the drawings that follow in this section, only **one** number will be shown for paired body parts (lungs, kidneys, arms, legs, shoulders, etc...).

FOOT REFLEX GUIDES

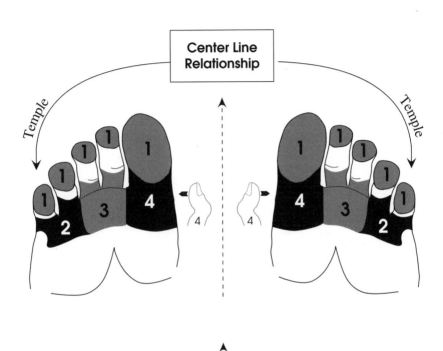

Center Line Relationship

Temple

Temple

Use your touch on the areas marked with numbers, and also the side of a numbered area where there's a thumb/arrow.

The little feet at the bottom of the pages of section C are to remind you about:

- the division areas (1-5)
- left and right, or
- the side of the foot shown.

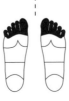

Right foot reflexes right side of body

Left foot reflexes left side of body

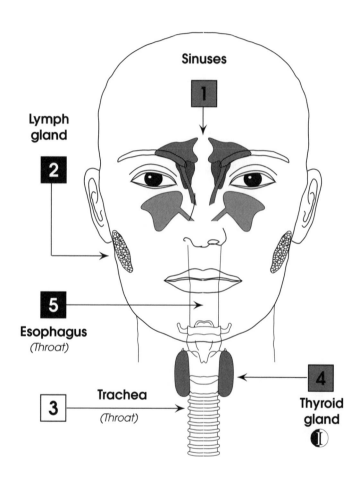

Sinuses

1

Lymph gland

2

5

Esophagus
(Throat)

Trachea
(Throat)

3

4

Thyroid gland

What we usually refer to as the **throat** is actually the top of two 'pipes' which lead to different places. The esophagus leads to the stomach. The trachea leads downwards to the lungs and also up into the nasal areas.

FOOT REFLEX GUIDES

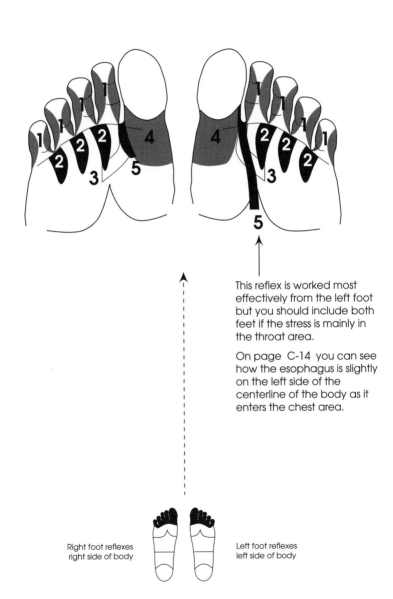

This reflex is worked most effectively from the left foot but you should include both feet if the stress is mainly in the throat area.

On page C-14 you can see how the esophagus is slightly on the left side of the centerline of the body as it enters the chest area.

Right foot reflexes right side of body

Left foot reflexes left side of body

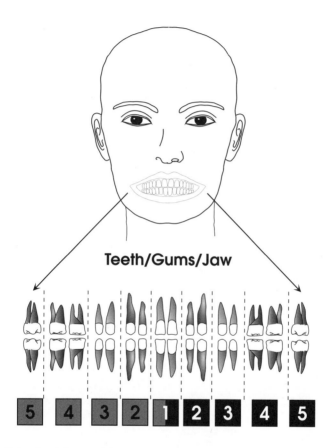

Teeth/Gums/Jaw

5 4 3 2 1 2 3 4 5

This chart is used to represent **zones** in the mouth that correspond to the reflexes on the toes. These are the famous zones that Dr. Fitzgerald did his work with, see pgs. B-16 &17.

The back of the mouth and molar teeth are in zone 5, and the center of the mouth and front teeth are in zone 1. Tooth, gum or jaw discomfort may show up as tender reflexes on the top side of the big toe (1) in addition to the related tooth to toe correspondence. So always check the big toe first and then the other toes (top and bottom of each toe).

FOOT REFLEX GUIDES

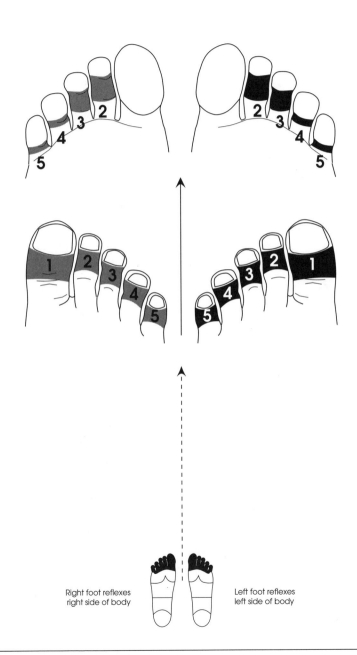

Right foot reflexes
right side of body

Left foot reflexes
left side of body

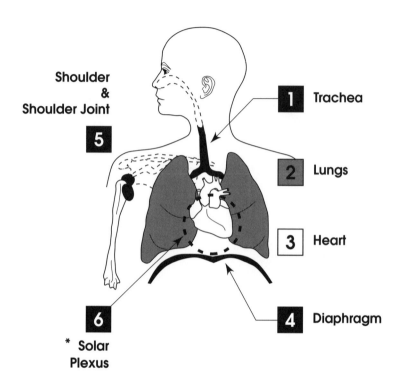

Shoulder & Shoulder Joint — **5**

1 Trachea

2 Lungs

3 Heart

4 Diaphragm

6 * Solar Plexus

* The solar plexus is a nerve complex which carries energy impulses to the heart, lungs and stomach. When there's a lot of physical or emotional stress, these functions of the body can also be quite stressed.

The best technique for this reflex is **continuous** thumb contact for 2-5 minutes or more on the reflex area. This "holding" technique is especially effective when working on others (see D-10 #5 for an illustration). Have the person be in a comfortable position, then hold the reflex area on both feet at the same time if possible. The relaxation effects will be optimized if you both **breathe** in deeply and exhale very slowly at the same rate while pressure is applied to the reflex.

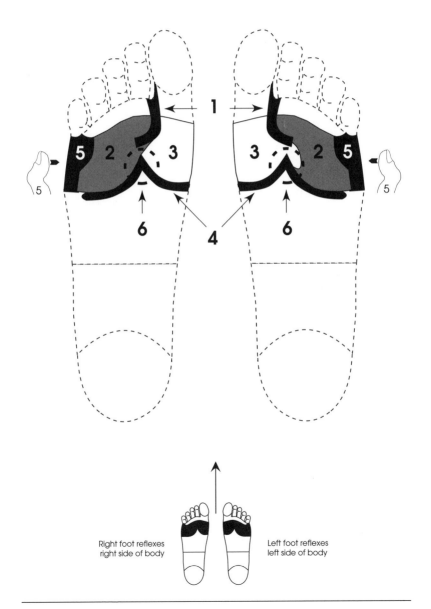

Right foot reflexes
right side of body

Left foot reflexes
left side of body

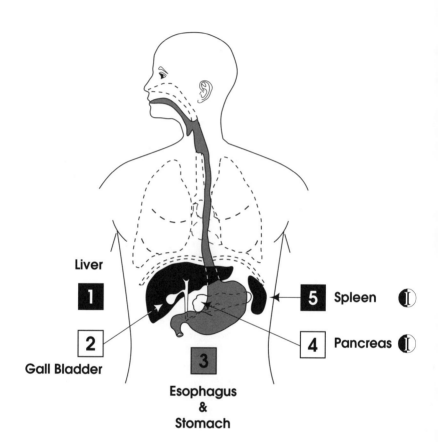

Liver

1

2

Gall Bladder

3

Esophagus
&
Stomach

5 Spleen

4 Pancreas

One of the functions of the spleen is to produce the type of white blood cells which fight infections. Reflexing for the spleen may help the natural immune functions of the body.

The pancreas contains a structure-(islets of Langerhans) that produce two hormone chemicals -(insulin & glucagon). These hormones assist immune functions through their balancing effects on blood sugar levels.

FOOT REFLEX GUIDES

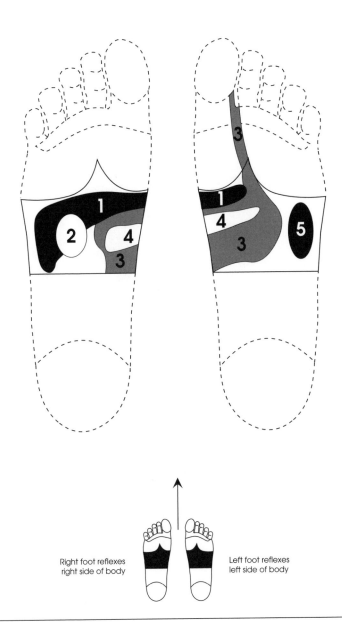

Right foot reflexes
right side of body

Left foot reflexes
left side of body

LOWER ABDOMEN & PELVIC AREA

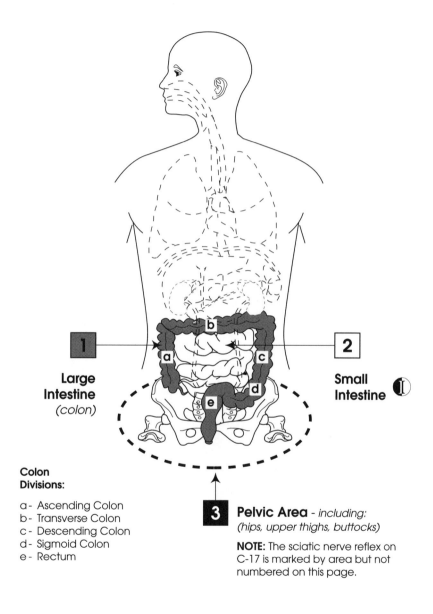

1 Large Intestine (colon)

2 Small Intestine

Colon Divisions:

a - Ascending Colon
b - Transverse Colon
c - Descending Colon
d - Sigmoid Colon
e - Rectum

3 **Pelvic Area** - including: (hips, upper thighs, buttocks)

NOTE: The sciatic nerve reflex on C-17 is marked by area but not numbered on this page.

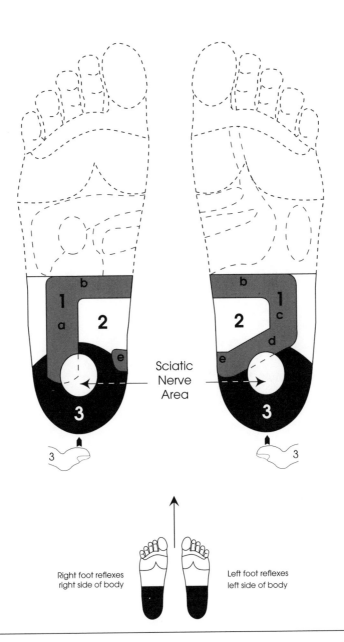

Sciatic
Nerve
Area

Right foot reflexes
right side of body

Left foot reflexes
left side of body

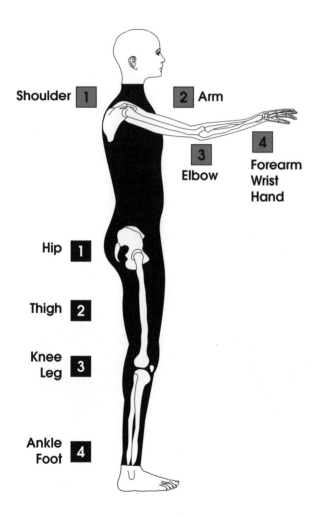

Shoulder **1**

2 Arm

3
Elbow

4
Forearm
Wrist
Hand

Hip **1**

Thigh **2**

Knee
Leg **3**

Ankle
Foot **4**

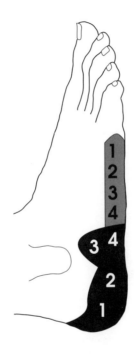

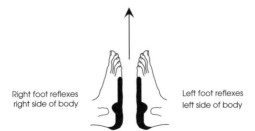

Right foot reflexes
right side of body

Left foot reflexes
left side of body

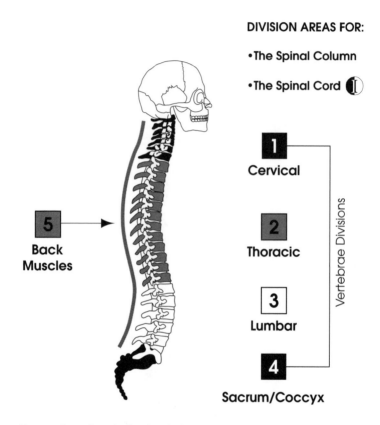

DIVISION AREAS FOR:

• The Spinal Column

• The Spinal Cord

1 Cervical

2 Thoracic

3 Lumbar

4 Sacrum/Coccyx

Vertebrae Divisions

5 Back Muscles

Energy **impulses** to the body travel through the spinal cord which is inside the spine. Stresses in spinal areas may often relate to problems in other areas of the body or vice-versa. For this reason, it's always good to **include reflexing for the spine,** whatever the situation may be.

The general rule of thumb is:

• If the stress is in the upper body, include reflexing for the cervicals and upper thoracic vertebrae.
• If the stress is in the torso area, include reflexing for the thoracic vertebrae.
• If the stress is in the pelvic area, include reflexing for the lumbar vertebrae and sacrum/coccyx.

FOOT REFLEX GUIDES

Back Muscles: *Muscles near the shoulder -* **(a)**

Muscles halfway across the back - **(b)**

Muscles near the spine - **(c)**

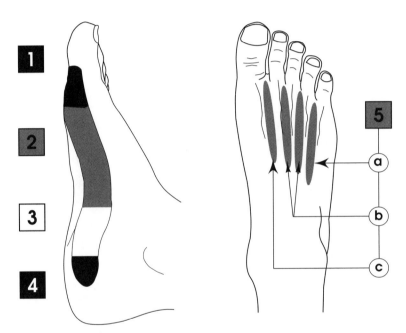

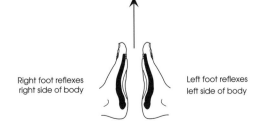

Right foot reflexes
right side of body

Left foot reflexes
left side of body

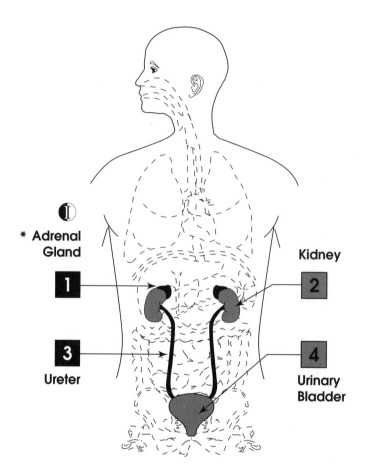

* **Adrenal Gland**

1

3

Ureter

Kidney

2

4

Urinary Bladder

* The adrenal glands are major structures to support the ability of the body to cope with stress. The adrenal glands produce adrenaline, which is important for balancing many body functions. Under prolonged stress, however, (quite a widespread situation these days), the body **accumulates** excessive adrenaline as toxins. The adrenals are labeled here along with the urinary system to highlight the importance of reflexing the adrenals and urinary functions together. This may help to flush toxins from the body, especially when extra water is taken.

FOOT REFLEX GUIDES

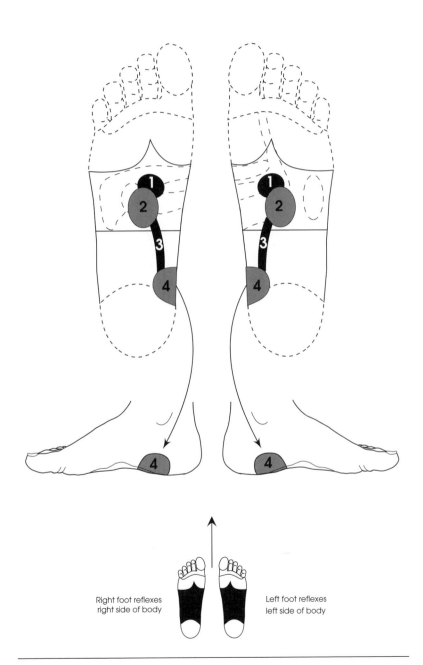

Right foot reflexes
right side of body

Left foot reflexes
left side of body

Combined Male and Female Representations

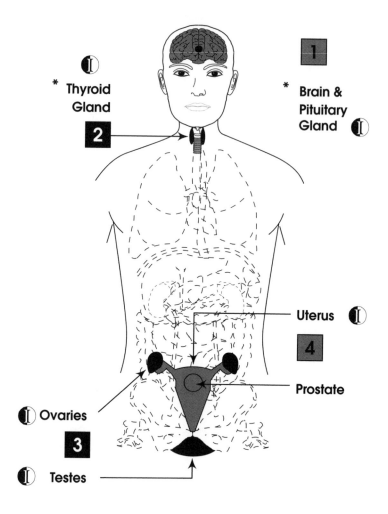

* Thyroid Gland

2

1

* Brain & Pituitary Gland

Uterus

4

Prostate

Ovaries

3

Testes

Procreation is fundamental to our livelihood. Reproduction is a complex process which includes spiritual, emotional and metabolic functions. As you may note, most of the associated reflex pathways shown here are supported by immune functions.

FOOT REFLEX GUIDES

Pituitary Gland
Reflexes

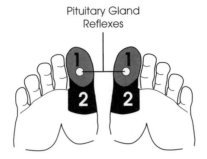

* The brain, pituitary and thyroid glands are "helper" reflexes for assisting general stress reduction and the functions of the reproductive systems.

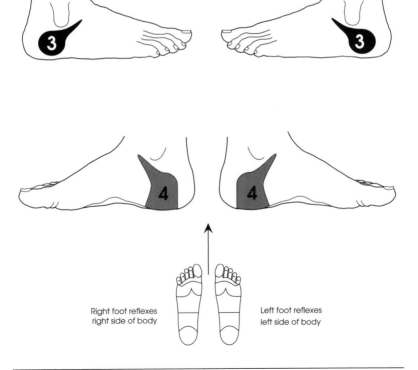

Right foot reflexes
right side of body

Left foot reflexes
left side of body

SUMMARY FOR REFLEXING

Can we see the forest for the trees? Well, sometimes it's difficult, unless we have a chance to pull back from the details, to adjust our vision so to speak. The charts on the facing page are to help you achieve this by summarizing **divisions** and **zones** together.

They're presented on separate feet as follows:

• **General Division Areas** **A** **B** **C** on the right foot.

• **Zones** A B C on the left foot.

The details aren't on these maps because they're meant to serve you for **navigating**. This is the one chart you should try to remember by heart!

But if you ever get too confused about reflexing, or caught up in the details of the maps, then remember the following **3 rules of 5's** :

1. There are **5** main general division areas.

2. There are **5** zones on each side of the center line of the body, relating to zones of the feet (and hands).

3. There are **5** considerations for reflexing effectively.

• **N**avigate the body, then the feet.

• **A**djust touch to the situation.

• **C**aterpillar action = micro-movements.

• **A**ttitude counts... and don't diagnose.

• **W**ork with tender reflexes, not just the ouch.

NACAW ...and five letters to help you remember these points.

DIVISION AREAS & ZONES

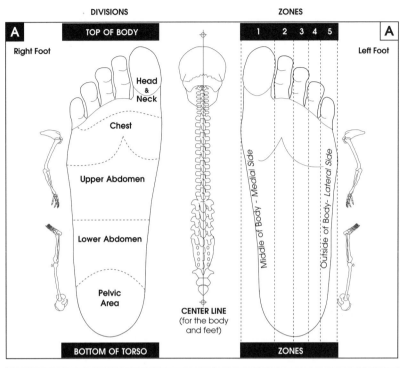

DIVISIONS

ZONES

A

TOP OF BODY

Right Foot

Head & Neck

Chest

Upper Abdomen

Lower Abdomen

Pelvic Area

BOTTOM OF TORSO

CENTER LINE
(for the body and feet)

1 2 3 4 5

A

Left Foot

Middle of Body - Medial Side

Outside of Body - Lateral Side

ZONES

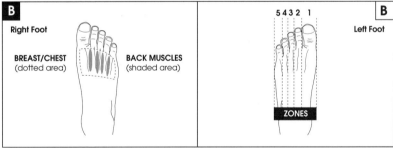

B

Right Foot

BREAST/CHEST
(dotted area)

BACK MUSCLES
(shaded area)

5 4 3 2 1

B

Left Foot

ZONES

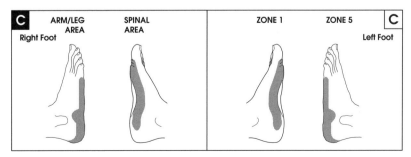

C

ARM/LEG AREA

SPINAL AREA

Right Foot

ZONE 1

ZONE 5

C

Left Foot

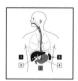

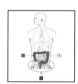

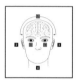

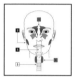

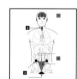

This page is meant to help you focus on some of the key points in Section C.
How many useful concepts or words come to mind?

D

**INFANT/CHILD
CARE**

Babies sometimes don't live their normal baby lives ... and then the whole family can suffer with the situation! Babies can't **communicate** their pains or discomforts very well, so parents often feel **helpless** with the problem. This helplessness may lead to even more stress for baby, and then the suffering goes around in a circle affecting everybody.

Reflexing for baby can be a wonderful help for **relaxing baby**, and working with their discomforts. It's also a way to relax and **support the love bond** between the parents and baby at a time of great need. Little ones are very receptive to natural healing energies, with love being the greatest of all. The techniques described in the following pages are based on letting this energy flow freely through your fingers... a very simple and tender experience for all.

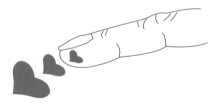

It should be obvious by now that the feet hold a few special considerations that relate to health. However, a few special considerations need to be taken when approaching the feet of an infant.

1. If you apply normal adult reflexing pressure to an infant, you probably won't have a chance to do it a second time.

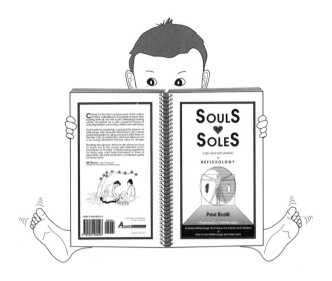

2. Reflexing for babies should be with a **light touch**, but not the tickling kind of touch (quick and scratch-like) which is something quite different.

3. By the age of 3, the reflexes can be worked with a little more pressure, but in all cases your best judge is the reaction of your child to your **loving touch**.

4. Until the age of 7, little ones usually **don't like** to have their toes reflexed! Nevertheless, some touch-play like "this little piggy" is a good way to get them used to some basic touch to the toes.

5. By getting your infant or child used to having the feet touched you'll be paving the way for **investing** in their heath... through their feet!

LOVE DE-STRESSES

1.   **Love energy** is a great healer, especially the love from a parent for a baby. Let this energy travel through your fingers while you're working with baby's feet. This is the most important guide for reflexing little ones. You will need to focus on relaxing yourself before approaching an infant. Holding **positive** thoughts about your ability to touch effectively are important and may be a key for helping you to relax while you reflex. Breathing in slowly and exhaling very slowly also helps to relax and focus on the matter at hand.

2.   There are three basic ways to approach little feet:
     a. A light **soothing** thumbwalk or stroking action **on the foot**
     b. A circular action **on** the foot - (finger or thumb) *
     c. A circular action **above** the foot - (finger or thumb) *

3.   If baby **pulls a foot away** from you at any time, work on the other one, then come back to the first one. Sometimes baby may only seem to want one foot worked on. This is normal and should be honored.

4.   For maximum benefit and relaxation, work the **whole foot**. Spend extra time in the area that corresponds to the stress that baby has. Do this by holding the area with light but constant pressure, or by making slow circular movements on the reflex area.

* *For more information on the circular technique, see 'Light Touch Reflex Action' - (**LTRA**) - in Section **Y** - pg. 3.*

5. Do as much as baby wants, or you feel you should do. The technique is very subtle, like the action of **caressing a flower petal**.

You might work for 5 minutes, or for 30 minutes or more. You can work as much as you want each day. You'll be helping baby to relax so that the "body harmony" can have a chance to sing its song more beautifully.

6. You might need to **distract** baby at times while reflexing, especially the first time. You might use a puppet or toy in one hand for this.

7. Talcum, body cream, lotion or oil may be used on the feet, but is **not necessary**.

8. You can reflex while baby is sleeping! You don't even have to touch the feet. Reflexes extend into the energy fields surrounding the feet (*the aura*). Just make very **slow circular movements** with your thumb or index finger 1/4"-1/2" in the air above the reflex. The direction of the circle rotations is not important. When you do this work, the little body might twitch a bit, which is normal. This is just an indication that energy pathways are being de-stressed.

9. The technique will be correct if your **attitude** is:
- to **focus on baby**, not the symptoms,
- to let the **fullness of your love** flow freely into the feet.

1. For this age group it's usually not necessary to distract the child while you work on the feet. The child will most likely **appreciate** and look forward to having the feet reflexed. There's no formal setting needed either. In the park, at the beach, while watching T.V. or reading can all be valid experiences for them. Children seem to understand the benefits of reflexing subconsciously. Share the concepts and drawings of this book with them. Communicate about the reflexes! They'll be fascinated. You won't just be helping them, you'll be **learning with them** since they just might understand it better and quicker than you.

2. This age group will love to have the feet reflexed **before going to sleep**. By this age, the mind is more conscious and active. Sleep can be disturbed more easily by the activities of the day, especially the negative or fearful stimuli. **Sleep is one third of a human life**, and we all know that there's plenty going on during sleep. So sleeping as relaxed as possible is pretty important. Reflexing on a regular basis may help with this. It's like an investment for their total well-being!

3. Reflexing for this age group can be a combination of the techniques for infants and adults. Since the child will be able to **communicate to you** in most cases, you should do what feels good for the child. Experiment with your touch to see what the child likes best. Sometimes they will actually tell you what kind of touch to apply to the feet. It might be little circular movements, or deeper work (thumbwalk) at other times.

4. Spend extra time on the reflex area for a particular discomfort (5-15 minutes). Try to work **as soon** as the discomfort is present, and continue until things start to relax in the body. When you reflex for a child it's quite useful to use a number scale to get feedback about the discomfort and how it eases.

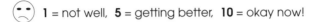 1 = not well, **5** = getting better, **10** = okay now!

Before reflexing, establish the reference number. Then as you continue reflexing, you can ask how much better things are getting.

5. If there are tender spots on the foot, the reflex correspondences can be explained to the child. They will very quickly learn the connection, and may even **tell you** where to reflex when they don't feel well. Many times just reflexing the **solar plexus** area might be asked for. This makes sense because it's a powerful reflex for promoting **relaxation** (see pg.C-12).

6. When the child's energy is low and there's more than one problem to deal with, reflex **both feet completely** (thumbwalk). It's quite normal for the child to fall into sleep during or after a session of 20 minutes or more. Sleep helps the healing!

7. There's no set time for reflexing for this age group. Do what's possible for you and your child.

ENCOURAGE A POSITIVE ATTITUDE TOWARDS THE FEET

Reflex maps for little ones are the same as for adults. Just smaller in area! An adult thumb or finger can cover a large part of a reflex area in many cases. So in addition to regular micro-movement techniques, there's another way to work the reflexes. **Hold** your **thumb** in place on a reflex area. Just the energy coming through your touch has an effect on the reflexes.

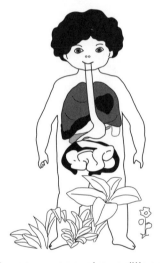

On the next page general conditions are shown: 1-5. Reflexing is illustrated overleaf for these discomforts. You can use the **holding** technique for **any area**, or reflex each foot one at a time. When a child can communicate, it's helpful to ask them to point to the area of the body that's under stress, or has pain. That way you can zero in on the right or left foot and the general foot reflex area. Remember that for adults, a tender reflex helps to navigate. With a child, however, the emphasis should be on working well **below** any **pain threshold** on the foot.

FOOT REFLEX GUIDES

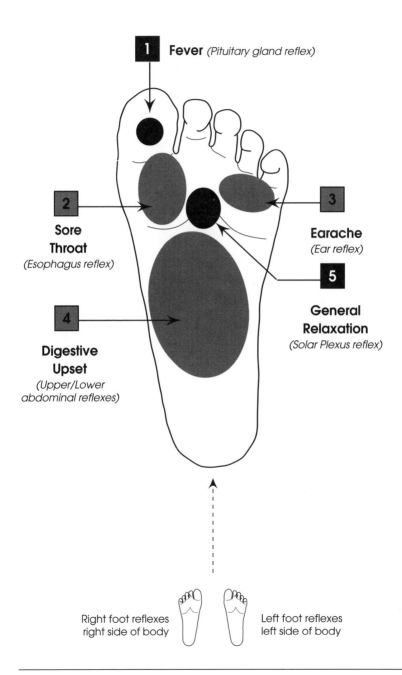

1 Fever *(Pituitary gland reflex)*

2 Sore Throat
(Esophagus reflex)

3 Earache
(Ear reflex)

4 Digestive Upset
(Upper/Lower abdominal reflexes)

5 General Relaxation
(Solar Plexus reflex)

Right foot reflexes right side of body

Left foot reflexes left side of body

1 **Fever** (reduction)

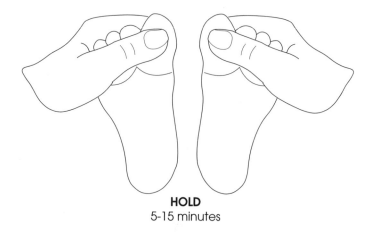

HOLD
5-15 minutes

5 **General Relaxation**
(asthma, vomiting, colic, hypertension, emotions, etc...)

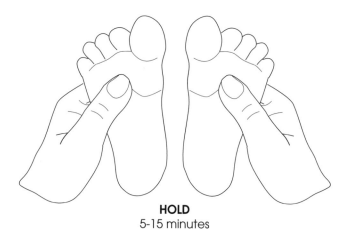

HOLD
5-15 minutes

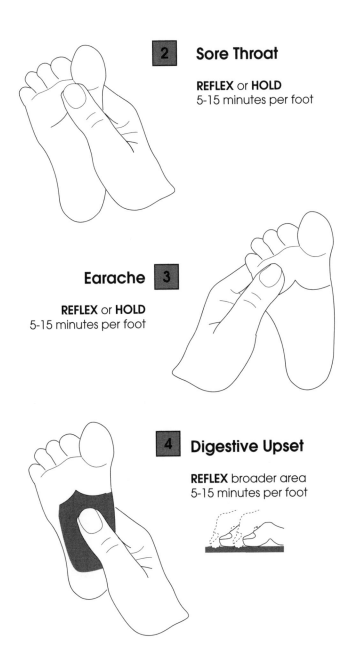

2 Sore Throat

REFLEX or **HOLD**
5-15 minutes per foot

Earache 3

REFLEX or **HOLD**
5-15 minutes per foot

4 Digestive Upset

REFLEX broader area
5-15 minutes per foot

Many books on reflexology include case studies about wonderful results experienced by people of all ages. Although such studies are purely anecdotal information (without scientific explanations), they have nevertheless motivated many people to explore reflexology for themselves. The following stories are presented in the same spirit, to encourage reflexing for those who cannot help themselves, infants and children.

Stress at the pool: A seven-year-old boy had been enjoying himself for hours at the pool on a sunny day. He suddenly suffered a digestive system upset and his mother wanted to take him home to attempt recovery. I asked permission to reflex his feet, explaining that an area of the foot might help reduce the stress his body was experiencing. The boy was excited about the fact that a spot on his foot might just help. I asked him to point to the area of his body that didn't feel good. It was in the lower abdominal area on the right side. I started reflexing lightly on the corresponding area of the right foot, asking if 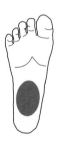 there was some pain there. He said there was but it was all right. Actually, I knew it before he told me since I'd noticed his wincing when the spot was reflexed. After about a long two minutes of reflexing his eyes lit up. He kindly said that the pain in his body had gone! He then ran off to his mother to report that he was okay and wanted to stay at the pool longer.

Digestive upset at a restaurant: A six-year-old girl was with a party of celebrating adults. After eating half of her dinner, the child wanted to go to the bathroom, feeling the urge to "pop her cookies". She did so and returned to her seat pale, weak and apparently ready to go home to rest. I was among the group and asked permission to take her foot in hand.

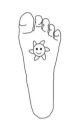

I asked where she felt the discomfort most. She pointed to her upper abdomen area on the left side. The corresponding area on the left foot was very tender to the touch, and a holding technique was used on the solar plexus reflex. I positioned her in her chair so that she could lean back and get a little comfortable. I explained that I would hold my thumb in the same spot and we would wait until things got better in her body. After 5 minutes of holding, the relaxation began to set in. After 10 minutes she fell asleep in the chair. She was covered to keep her warm, and the party continued. Half an hour later she awoke in good spirits and ready to rejoin the celebration.

Sick at home: A five-year-old boy developed severe digestive disturbances with vomiting and associated weaknesses and fever. The child was made as comfortable as possible in bed. Each foot was reflexed completely for 20 minutes.

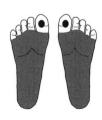

...continued next page

The toes were excluded, but holding the pituitary reflexes at the same time on the big toes (3 minutes) was included to finish off the reflexing. The child grew more and more relaxed as the first foot was reflexed. By the time the second foot was being reflexed he was almost ready to sleep. A deep sleep followed the work on the feet and the child awoke 3 hours later. Having recovered from the disturbance, the child was happy to resume normal activities.

Pain at school: My daughter, at the age of 6, developed considerable ear pain while at school . She asked her teacher to call me, wanting her feet reflexed for the pain. I met her and could have reflexed at school but decided to take her home to work on her feet. The pain was in her left ear. Before starting to reflex I 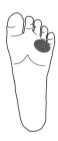 asked her how bad the pain was on the 1 to 10 scale. A 10, she said! Gentle pressure was applied to the ear reflex of the left foot. It was very tender, she winced. We decided to use the holding technique. After holding for five minutes she said the ear was hurting less. We continued for another five minutes and she said the ear felt better still, now a 5 on the scale. Holding continued for another ten minutes, and the pain disappeared and did not return. She resumed her normal activities without any discomforts.

These kinds of stories could continue... and **they should** don't you think!

If there's one message to gain from the pages of this section, it's to have the **compassion** and **courage** to reach out to little ones in their times of need. It's natural for adults to coddle, stroke, rock, hug and kiss infants and children when they have pain, discomfort or sickness. So reach out to them with this tender experience. Communicate to them through the feet. Let them guide you as you learn together about the benefits of this safe and effective touch technique. Yes, it takes time... but adults or parents **benefit** at the same time since their own livelihoods are often linked to the distressed child's comfort level.

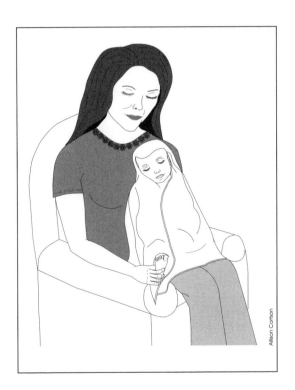

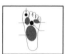

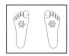

This page is meant to help you focus on some of the key points in Section D.
How many useful concepts or words come to mind?

FOOT CHARTS

W

**FOOT
CHARTS**

Color coding is a great way for the brain to remember things. Have fun with your coloring pencils or felt-tips in this section by bringing the **pages to life**! Use lighter colors for the larger reflex areas, and darker colors for the smaller areas, especially if they're marked off inside other areas.

• The first part (**4-13**) **reinforces** and **expands** on what you learned about reflexes in Sections A-D. Some of the reflexes are grouped together in new ways to broaden your understanding. Match the **small letters** of the headings a to a matching reflex a location(in dotted lines). Use the same color for both. The reflex may be on both feet or only on one.

• The second part (**14-20**) gives you space to **practice** what you've learned, or a place for records of your own experiences.

Above all...
Have fun!

Indicates reflexing an area on the side of the foot.

Specifies glands or structures involved in immune functions.

8 colored pencils or felt-tips are needed for this section.

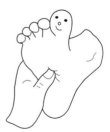

BRAIN a

The organ which controls most of the body's activities. It receives information, and sends messages through chemical and electrical activity. • Stressed on a daily basis!

EARS b

The organs of hearing and balance. • They may frequently be a site of discomfort for children or for anyone suffering from sinus congestion or a bout with a common cold.

EYES c

The organs of sight which send nervous impulses to the brain when stimulated by light rays. • Stressed on a daily basis, the eyes may be the site of a variety of discomforts or imbalances.

d PITUITARY

A gland within the brain which secretes hormones into the bloodstream. The master control for the immune system, stimulates other glands. • An excellent stress reducing reflex for most situations.

e FOREHEAD

This head area contains sinuses and the frontal lobe of the brain which is the site of mental activities. • This reflex is effective for reducing pain associated with many common situations.

f NECK

The neck area is like a tunnel through which all kinds of communication travels back and forth from the brain/head area to the body. • A site of stress for many people on a daily basis.

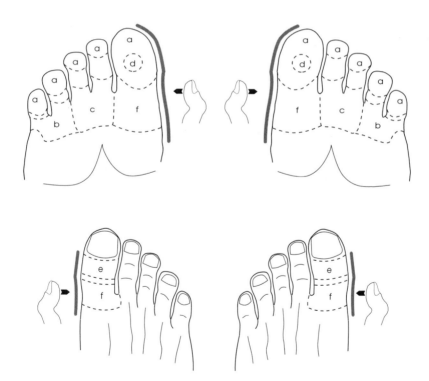

RIGHT FOOT   LEFT FOOT

EUSTACHIAN TUBE 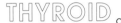 a

An air-filled tube that keeps air pressure equal on both sides of the eardrum. •This tube may become blocked creating ear discomfort. Reflexing may normalize the situation.

d SINUSES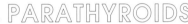

Air-filled cavities that reduce the weight of the skull. When irritated they swell, create pressure & block drainage.• Stressed with colds, allergies, headaches, tooth/jaw pain, and breathing difficulties.

TRACHEA b

The tube through which air passes on its way to and from the lungs. The upper part is also referred to as the throat. • A site of stress with colds, breathing difficulties, and loss of voice.

e LYMPH GLANDS

The site of disease-fighting cells that filter and recycle body fluids. • The lymph glands in the neck area may be a site of stress associated with imbalances in the head area or the common cold.

THYROID c ❶

A gland in the neck area producing several hormones regulating growth, metabolism, sexual development and overall immune functions. • A major reflex for promoting vitality.

❶ f PARATHYROIDS

Four small glands lying under the thyroid regulating the levels of calcium and phosphate in the blood. • May be stressed due to mental or physical fatigue.

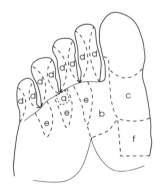
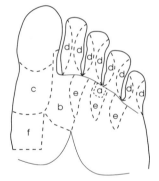

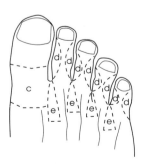
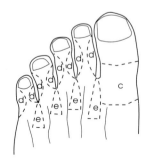

RIGHT FOOT

LEFT FOOT

ZONES

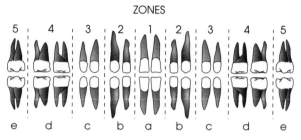

Dr. Fitzgerald developed the zone theory of reflex work with a lot of attention given to the zones of the face, and especially the teeth. He discovered that applying pressure to fingers and toes in the related zones produced an anesthetic effect to the corresponding tooth area.

In addition, it seems that nerve pathways to and from the teeth are linked energetically to the rest of the body, along the zones. So it's possible for a zone problem in the mouth to be linked to energetic imbalances anywhere along the zone. For this reason, it's a good idea to check the whole zone of the foot for additional tender areas other than for the specific tooth reflex. Do this by reflexing all the way down from under a toe to the base of the foot in a band about the width of the toe.

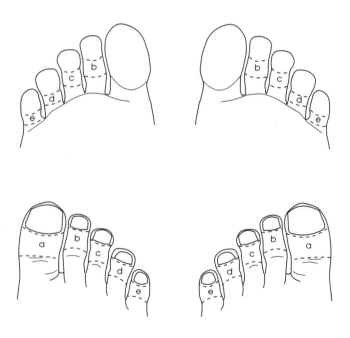

RIGHT FOOT   LEFT FOOT

NECK LINE a

The area from the base of the neck to the shoulders which includes the collar bone. • Tension in this area may accumulates on a daily basis due to poor posture and/or mental stresses.

DIAPHRAGM b

A sheet of muscular tissue which separates the chest from the upper abdomen•When there's a lot of emotional stress or breathing difficulties, this area may carry a lot of tension.

SOLAR PLEXUS c

Also referred to as the midbrain of the body, a nerve complex coming off the spinal cord that carries electrical impulses to the heart, lungs and stomach. • A major reflex for relaxing the body.

d HEART

A muscular organ that pumps blood around the body through blood vessels, carrying nutrients (energy) to all parts of the body. • A site of stress for emotional and/or physical imbalances.

e LUNGS

The two main breathing organs where gases (oxygen & carbon dioxide) are exchanged. •A site of stress for emotional and physical imbalances including asthma and common colds.

f BREAST AREA

This area holds the mammary glands (females), that produce milk. • A site of stress for emotional and physical imbalances especially during menstruation, pregnancy and infant care.

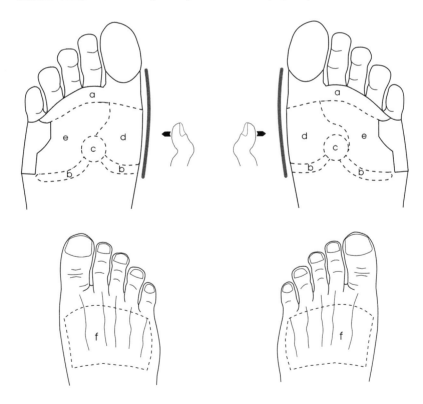

RIGHT FOOT   LEFT FOOT

LIVER a

The liver has hundreds of functions including secretion of bile for digestion, storing vitamins & iron, making blood proteins and filtering blood. • May be stressed daily due to improper diet/ life-style.

PANCREAS b

The pancreas produces digestive juices that continue breaking down food passing from the stomach into the duodenum (first part of the small intestine). Also the site of production of insulin.

GALL BLADDER c

A sac which stores bile (made in the liver) in a concentrated form until it is needed for digestion. • An imbalance of the gall bladder may lead to radiating pain up to the right shoulder area.

d STOMACH

A muscular sac that mixes and churns food, saliva, mucus and digestive chemicals. • A common site of stress especially when meals are eaten too quickly or the food is not fresh.

e ESOPHAGUS

The tube that links the mouth to the stomach. • May be stressed or irritated due to vomiting, acid conditions of the stomach, belching, and the lodging of food particles.

f SPLEEN

An organ that stores emergency supplies of red blood cells and produces the type of white blood cells which fight infections. • Reflexing may help balance anemic conditions and fight infections.

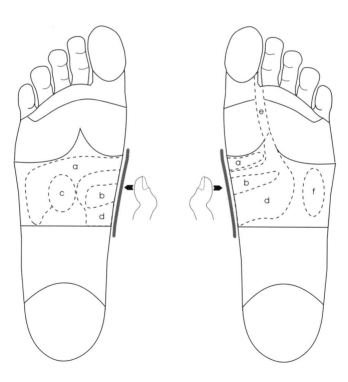

RIGHT FOOT   LEFT FOOT

S. INTESTINE a ⟨I⟩

A long tube where food is further broken down after leaving the stomach so that it can be used as energy by the rest of the body• May be the site of imbalance due to improper diet/ life-style.

L. INTESTINE b

Also called the colon, a thick tube receiving waste from the small intestine. It's main function is to remove water from the feces. • May be the site of imbalance due to improper diet/ life-style.

RECTUM c

The final section of the colon which stores the end products of digestion until they can be eliminated. • May be the site of stress due to improper diet/ life-style.

d APPENDIX

A small sac at the begining of the colon. Our ancestors might have needed it more than we do to filter toxins from unrefined foods. • May become inflamed leading to surgical removal.

e ILEOCECAL

A 'one-way valve' regulating the flow of digestion from the s. intestine into the colon. • An important reflex for digestion or imbalances of the body that produce excessive mucous discharge.

f SIGMOID FLEXURE

A bend in the last part of the large intestine (on the left side of the body) before the rectum. • Intestinal gases tend to get trapped in this area, and reflexing for the sigmoid flexure may have amazing (releasing) results!

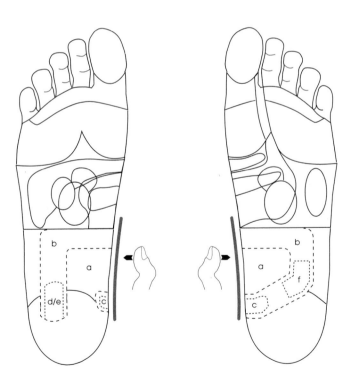

RIGHT FOOT   LEFT FOOT

PELVIC REFLEXES

OVARIES-TESTES a

Female/male (gonads). Apart from respective reproductive functions, they're sites of hormone production for both sexes. •Sites of stress for a variety of reasons since their functions are central to daily life.

UTERUS-PROSTATE b

The uterus is a hollow organ inside which a fetus is held. The prostate helps regulate the flow of semen and urine. • May be sites of stress for a variety of reasons - for women on a regular basis after puberty - for men later in life.

SCIATIC NERVE c

A large nerve which supplies energy impulses to the legs and feet. • May be a site of energy blockage, stress or inflammation due to a combination of physical and emotional situations, or trauma to the spine.

d BUTTOCKS

More commonly referred to by 3 or 4 letter words, a site of stress & tension for many. Does it always sit in a comfortable position?

e BLADDER

A muscular sac that stores urine until it can be released from the body, usually by conscious mechanisms. • May be a site of stress or inflammation due to a variety of (aggravating) physical or emotional situations.

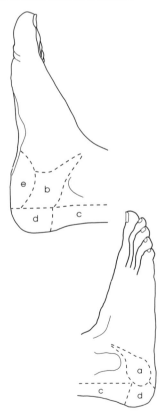
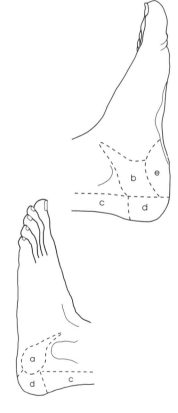

RIGHT FOOT   LEFT FOOT

SHOULDER/ARM a

The shoulder is a broad structure which attaches the arm to the body and has a ball and socket joint allowing the arm to move in all directions. • Site of tension or injury due to life-style and even mental stress.

ELBOW b

The hinge joint connecting the arm to the forearm. • A frequent site of traumas due to accidents or sports-related injuries. Tennis elbow anyone? This reflex may be very effective for addressing such a situation.

WRIST/HAND c

The wrists and hands are active all the time during our waking hours. •Micro-movements of the fingers and wrist while using computer keyboards is a serious stress syndrome these days.

d HIP/THIGH

The hip bone's connected to the thigh bone - so the song goes! • A frequent site of traumas due to accidents to the bones or muscles (hamstrings, on backside of thigh).

e KNEE/LEG

The knee is a hinge joint connecting the thigh to the leg. • The knee is a common site of trauma or inflammation. This reflex may be very effective for addressing such a situation.

f ANKLE/FOOT

The ankle connects the foot to the leg, and the foot allows us to stand upright. • Together they bear the weight of the body... and as you may now appreciate... life itself!

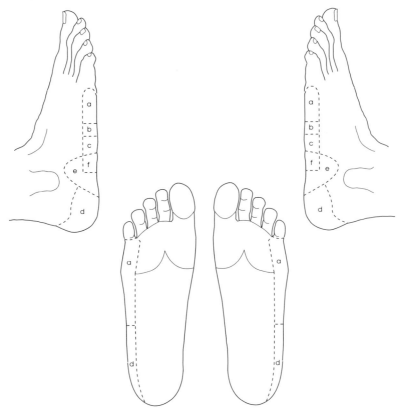

RIGHT FOOT

LEFT FOOT

CERVICAL _a

The first 7 vertebrae of the spine supporting the neck
• Common site of tension, pain or injury.

THORACIC _b

The next 12 vertebrae of the spine supporting the middle back & ribs. • Common site of tension.

LUMBAR _c

The 5 vertebrae of the lower back. • Common site of tension due to life-style, PMS, injury or lack of exercise.

SACRUM/COCCYX _d

The sacrum/coccyx are fused bone structures at the bottom of the spine. Ever have something hit you on the tailbone?

_e MUSCLES

The back muscles near the shoulder.

_f MUSCLES

Muscles halfway across the back.

_g MUSCLES

Muscles near the spine.

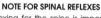

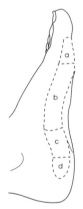

NOTE FOR SPINAL REFLEXES

Reflexing for the spine is important and beneficial because it's not just relaxing the vertebrae, but the broader areas that include:
• the spinal cord inside the spine, and
• the peripheral nerves that come out from the spine to carry electrical impulses to the organs, glands and structures that the nerves travel to.

NOTE FOR MUSCLE REFLEXES

These reflexes are more important for adults than for children, perhaps due to life-style tensions, aggravating posture and... carrying the weight of the world on our backs !#?

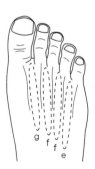

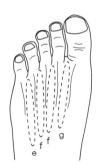

RIGHT FOOT

LEFT FOOT

REFLEXES FOR **HARMONY**

BRAIN a

We think... therefore we are. And it's said that we only use about $1/10$ of its potential! Keep it relaxed.

NECK AREA b

A site of pain, for ourselves... or maybe even for others! It also supports the skull & brain (see above).

ADRENALS c

The fight or flight glands. We battle with this seesaw situation all the time, whether we know it or not.

KIDNEYS d

The kidneys filter our blood and waste fluids. Would you swim in a pool that didn't have good filters?

e SPLEEN

Kind of like the emergency gas tank. It's there just in case.... but for our blood.

f GONADS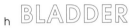

One of the functions of these structures is often central to everything these days!

g SPINE

A spine rub feels wonderful... but reflexing for the spine balances energy pathways.

h BLADDER

And drinking plenty of fresh water will help flush the waste products out of there!

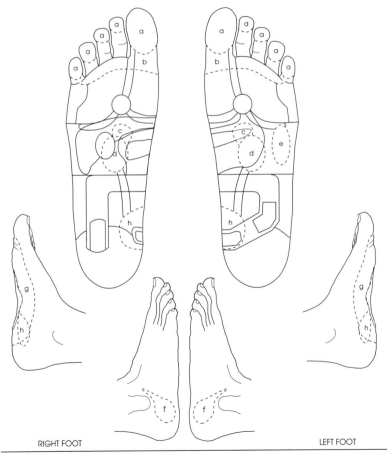

RIGHT FOOT   LEFT FOOT

FOOT

Name _____ Date _____

_____

_____

_____

_____

_____

_____

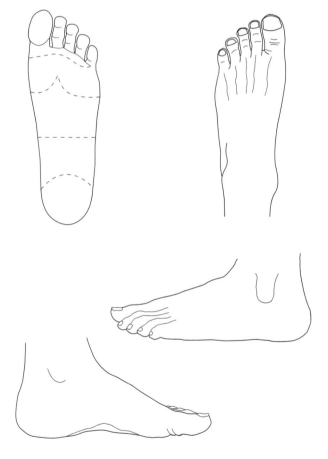

LEFT FOOT

_____
_____
_____
_____
_____
_____
_____
_____
_____

RIGHT FOOT

FOOT

Name _____ Date _____

_____

_____

_____

_____

_____

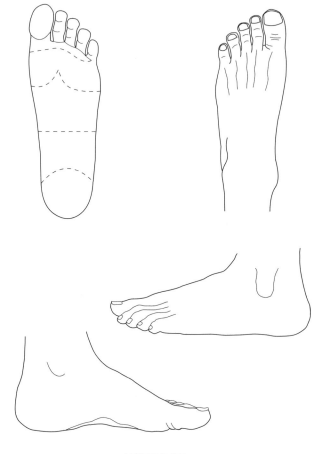

LEFT FOOT

_____
_____
_____
_____
_____
_____
_____
_____
_____
_____

RIGHT FOOT

Name

Date

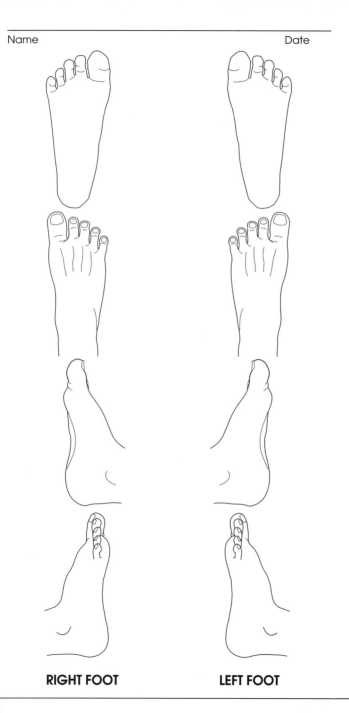

RIGHT FOOT　　　**LEFT FOOT**

LITTLE FOOT NOTES 2

Name _____

Date _____

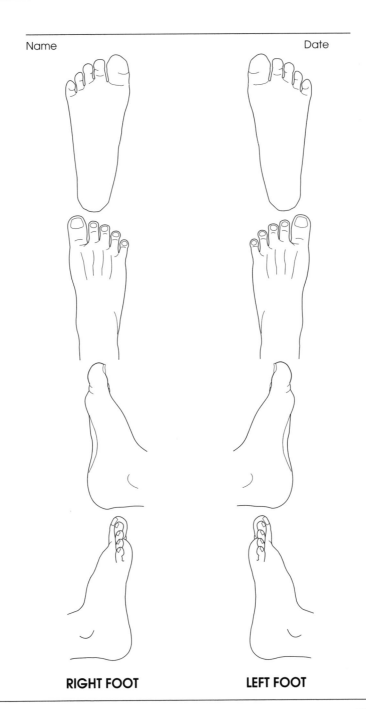

RIGHT FOOT **LEFT FOOT**

Name

Date

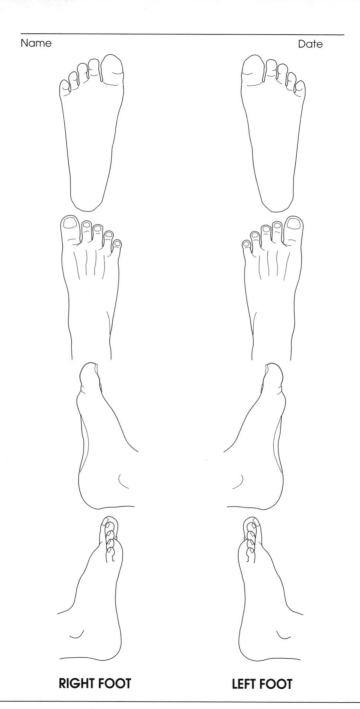

RIGHT FOOT   **LEFT FOOT**

WORD GAMES

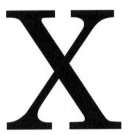

X

**WORD
GAMES**

CAUTIONS - CROSSWORD

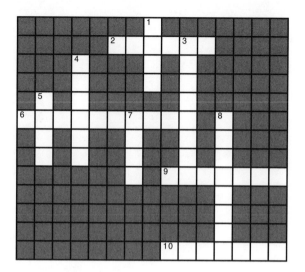

Across

2 Never reflex over open
_ _ _ _ _ _, cuts or bruises.
Washing your hands is appropriate before and after reflexing for someone besides yourself.

6 A lighter pressure should be used if a person is taking a quantity of _ _ _ _ _ _ _ _ _ _.

9 Only _ _ _ _ _ _ _ professionals are legally licensed to diagnose. Just because a reflex area is tender doesn't mean somethings wrong in the body.

10 It's important to adjust the pressure of your touch when reflexing for others, especially for the young and _ _ _ _ _ _ _ since their sensitivities may be more delicate due to their ages.

Down

1 Open _ _ _ _ in the skin should not be reflexed over.

3 Only medical professionals are licensed to _ _ _ _ _ _ _ _.

4 It can be black and blue and quite tender to the touch. If you must reflex over such an area use a light and tender touch!

5 Physically or emotionally _ _ _ _ individuals, as well as the elderly and children should be reflexed with a lighter touch than the average person.

7 You should never use one of these when reflexing someone besides yourself.

8 Reflexing over large exposed _ _ _ _ _ _ _ _ veins is not recommended since the pressure may aggravate the already stressed condition of the veins.

CAUTIONS - WORD SEARCH

2

M	L	B	R	U	I	S	E	K	L	A
D	E	O	Y	R	V	W	A	O	N	V
I	I	D	O	T	J	E	N	G	X	A
A	N	L	I	T	W	G	L	S	Q	R
G	F	G	M	C	N	E	K	O	U	I
N	A	P	B	A	A	D	P	N	P	C
O	N	E	I	E	X	T	N	R	T	O
S	T	L	S	N	U	J	I	U	H	S
E	S	T	M	W	K	R	P	O	O	E
W	U	Y	L	R	E	D	L	E	N	W
C	Z	U	N	E	R	D	L	I	H	C

Search for the **words**: forwards, backwards, diagonally.

TOOL
CUTS
BRUISE
ANGLE
DIAGNOSE

WEAK
WOUND
VARICOSE
LONGNAILS
MEDICATION

ELDERLY   CHILDREN   INFANT

3

S	T	L	I	C	E	N	S	E	D	N	D	M
U	Y	E	C	D	Z	Q	Y	M	J	S	T	P
S	G	H	N	E	Z	N	J	O	H	S	R	Y
Y	W	O	K	D	V	O	A	C	U	O	L	Q
G	E	C	S	R	E	I	U	J	F	N	S	H
N	S	T	U	K	O	R	T	E	O	R	H	X
I	O	R	V	X	X	W	S	C	Q	Y	A	M
X	N	T	Q	P	O	S	X	A	E	G	H	O
E	G	E	Y	Z	I	E	A	M	R	F	I	H
L	A	R	C	O	L	N	W	G	O	T	F	C
F	I	C	N	F	V	X	Y	Y	I	S	X	E
E	D	A	E	A	D	M	C	Z	N	C	T	E
R	L	R	M	G	D	L	A	C	I	D	E	M

These **words** make **phrases**, search: forwards, backwards, diagonally.

ONLY   MEDICAL   PROFESSIONAL   LICENSED   DIAGNOSE

MOST   EFFECTIVE   REFLEXING   JUST   WORK   TENDER   REFLEX   EXTRA

4

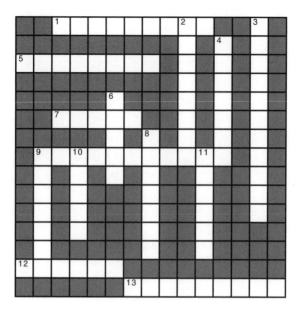

Across

1 This valve connects the small intestines to the large intestines and prevents backflow of fecal matter into the small intestines.

5 This organ produces insulin & chemicals to further break down food after leaving the stomach.

7 The largest organ inside the body - mostly on the right side.

9 The midbrain of the body.

12 Top part of the esophagus.

13 A muscular tissue which separates the chest from the upper abdomen area.

Down

2 It's in the lower right abdomen area. It can rupture and need surgical intervention.

3 The small sac which stores the bile produced in the liver.

4 The main organs of fluid excretion which filter the blood and regulate the level and contents of body fluids.

6 It pumps blood and is the strongest muscle of the body.

8 Urine is stored here until it can be expelled from the body.

9 The main site of digestion. It's about the size of a closed fist in most people when empty.

10 The main organs of respiration found in the chest.

11 Tube which carries urine from a kidney to the urinary bladder.

INTERNAL ORGANS - WORD SEARCH

5

S	T	L	J	X	I	D	N	E	P	P	A	R
T	U	A	U	H	C	A	M	O	T	S	E	G
E	B	X	O	N	T	G	K	I	E	T	A	K
L	L	E	E	R	G	Q	X	I	E	L	S	I
A	A	Y	S	L	H	S	A	R	L	U	P	D
C	D	W	R	B	P	T	U	B	T	K	D	N
E	D	O	H	E	E	R	L	L	X	J	H	E
C	E	I	E	J	Z	A	A	T	V	M	H	Y
O	R	T	E	R	D	O	Q	L	R	V	M	S
E	Z	R	E	D	U	G	X	S	O	A	X	A
L	P	V	E	W	W	Y	D	S	M	S	E	D
I	I	R	P	S	A	E	R	C	N	A	P	H
L	D	I	A	P	H	R	A	G	M	A	X	L

Search for the **words**: forwards, backwards, diagonally.

HEART
THROAT
PANCREAS
APPENDIX
ILEOCECAL

LIVER
LUNGS
URETER
KIDNEYS
BLADDER

DIAPHRAGM   GALLBLADDER   SOLARPLEXUS   STOMACH

6

S	C	E	H	O	E	E	P	A	Z	N	M
T	N	O	D	L	R	C	T	G	O	S	B
O	O	R	L	I	P	G	K	T	Y	O	E
M	T	D	Q	O	S	T	Z	M	D	Q	J
A	S	G	C	T	N	T	M	Y	N	N	E
C	A	C	Y	V	O	E	F	G	N	I	D
H	M	C	V	K	T	O	S	E	K	D	I
N	E	O	Q	R	N	N	F	E	L	F	S
P	A	M	I	O	E	K	Q	U	L	H	N
P	D	C	E	Y	X	O	B	T	J	O	I
W	A	R	S	P	L	E	E	N	U	J	S
L	A	S	I	G	M	O	I	D	D	C	Q

These **words** make **phrases**, search: forwards, backwards, diagonally.

SPLEEN   STOMACH   SIGMOID   COLON   AREON   LEFTSIDE

BODY   NOT   SYMMETRICAL   INSIDE   FOOT   SOLES   NOTSAME

7

[Crossword grid with numbered cells: 1, 2, 3, 4, 5, 6, 7, 8, 9, 10, 11, 12, 13]

Across

1 The _ _ _ bone's connected to the thigh bone.......

3 Has upper and lower parts connected by hinge joints and seats the teeth.

5 Has a ball and socket pivot which allows you to move your arm above your head.

8 The last member of the spine also known as the tail bone.

9 The 5 vertebrae of the lower back just above the sacrum.

12 The hinge joint connecting the thigh to the leg bones.

13 The 7 vertebrae which make up the neck and support the skull.

Down

1 It has a thumb and 4 fingers.

2 One of what you walk on.

4 The hinge joint connecting the forearm bones to the hand. This is the site of carpal tunnel syndrome, a common stress for many people these days.

5 The 5 fused vertebrae at the base of the spinal column.

6 The _ _ _ _ protect the inner cavity of the chest and upper abdomen.

7 The 12 vertebrae of the middle back which support the ribs.

10 The joint connecting the two leg bones to the foot. It often gets traumatized or bruised and reflexing for this may be very beneficial.

11 The skeletal casing which protects the brain.

BONES & JOINTS - WORD SEARCH

8

C	H	L	S	R	E	G	N	I	F	B
C	O	I	L	H	T	W	A	J	O	C
I	E	C	N	U	T	H	C	N	H	R
C	H	E	C	G	K	S	E	J	C	A
A	C	C	N	Y	E	S	I	E	I	B
R	E	E	K	K	X	J	R	R	I	M
O	O	I	R	B	A	V	O	H	W	U
H	T	I	M	N	I	H	F	I	I	L
T	B	U	K	C	A	I	W	O	N	P
S	H	L	A	N	T	C	I	R	O	T
T	E	L	D	S	A	C	R	U	M	T

Search for the **words**: forwards, backwards, diagonally.

ANKLE
BONE
CERVICAL
COCCYX
FINGERS
FOOT

HINGEJOINT
HAND
HIP
JAW
KNEE
LUMBAR

RIBS   SACRUM   SKULL   THORACIC   THUMB   TOE   WRIST

9

R	W	M	I	D	D	L	E	V	T	E
U	K	H	U	P	P	E	R	A	N	C
W	O	E	I	Q	J	O	I	I	E	Q
N	X	Y	A	C	L	L	P	R	L	R
O	Y	N	O	R	H	S	V	I	O	A
I	C	G	N	D	B	I	U	S	W	B
S	C	V	I	C	C	E	P	B	E	M
N	O	L	A	A	K	N	T	A	R	U
E	C	R	L	A	W	L	X	R	R	L
T	R	S	S	A	C	R	U	M	E	T
Y	T	H	O	R	A	C	I	C	V	V

These **words** make:

a. phrase
b. word match-ups,

Search: forwards, backwards, diagonally.

a.

WHICH   PART   SPINE   VERTEBRAE   DOYOU   CARRY   TENSION

b.

UPPER   MIDDLE   LOWER   TAIL

CERVICALS   THORACIC   LUMBAR   SACRUM   COCCYX

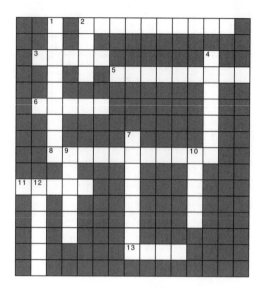

Across

2 This doctor is credited with the founding of what is considered modern reflexology.

3 Five _ _ _ _ _ on each side of the body centerline travel down into the hands and feet.

5 When your thumb moves like a caterpillar, its a _ _ _ _ _ _ _ _ _.

6 You can practice reflexing on them and be relaxing the body. They have full maps of the body very similar to the foot maps.

8 Touch pressure should be adjusted for each person since _ _ _ _ _ _ _ _ _ _ _ differs for each individual.

11 Dr. _ _ _ _ _ is credited with the horizontal division of the foot.

13 The outer _ _ _ _ may also be used for reflexing. Have maps resembling a shape of the body.

Down

1 A main theory of reflexology proposes that _ _ _ _ _ _ _ _ _ of energy are reduced so that the body can balance itself.

2 They carry you through life!

4 Body _ _ _ _ _ _ _ is like a symphony orchestra.

7 Your positive _ _ _ _ _ _ _ _ towards touching is as important as the touch itself.

9 It surrounds us and is the basis for all life in the universe.

10 If you aren't sure about your _ _ _ _ _, it's best to start off lightly, and gradually apply more pressure.

12 An American woman credited with the modern day pioneering and promotion of the mirror image concept of foot reflexology.

WELL BEING / DIS-EASE WORD SEARCH

11

G	S	L	I	V	E	F	O	O	D	N	R	W
Y	W	M	B	A	L	A	N	C	E	Y	A	C
S	I	C	I	S	Q	K	J	W	O	T	O	H
N	E	Y	I	L	U	L	D	E	E	M	D	O
E	V	N	L	J	E	O	C	R	P	D	S	N
R	I	O	A	V	K	L	E	A	H	L	Z	E
A	T	M	P	G	P	N	S	T	Q	Q	S	S
C	I	R	M	N	G	S	W	C	R	Q	J	T
T	S	A	G	V	I	T	X	L	N	U	D	Y
O	O	H	J	O	W	G	I	B	Q	A	O	R
O	P	Y	N	J	X	G	O	L	R	S	E	C
F	O	O	P	T	I	M	I	S	M	K	I	L
J	E	X	E	R	C	I	S	E	F	A	D	M

Search for the **words**: forwards, backwards, diagonally.

BALANCE
EXERCISE
FOOTCARE
HARMONY
HONESTY

LEAN
SMILE
POSITIVE
WATER
LIVEFOOD

COMPASSION JOY OPTIMISM COURTEOUS

12

X	D	Y	E	G	A	K	C	O	L	B	F	N
S	S	W	A	U	D	N	I	A	P	E	O	A
F	E	T	O	Z	C	M	D	W	A	H	T	U
O	A	V	R	T	K	O	A	R	O	Y	E	F
O	V	G	R	E	W	N	J	P	Y	I	N	D
T	D	F	G	E	S	C	E	R	U	W	S	O
P	M	Z	T	R	N	S	A	V	N	D	I	O
A	L	P	X	V	E	T	T	V	K	Q	O	F
I	C	W	X	N	N	S	K	D	X	N	N	D
N	P	F	W	E	O	N	S	J	I	Q	W	A
S	L	O	D	R	T	E	C	I	T	G	Q	E
Z	R	E	F	P	S	D	A	W	O	Y	I	D
F	S	I	V	U	R	E	D	D	C	N	I	R

Search for the **words**: forwards, backwards, diagonally.

FEAR
PAIN
NERVES
FROWN
TENSION

RIGID
STRESS
NOHOPE
FOOTPAIN
BLOCKAGE

AGGRESSION SEDENTARY DEADFOOD

PUZZLE SOLUTIONS

1 — CAUTIONS

Across:
2. WOUNDS
6. MEDICATION
9. MEDICAL
10. ELDERLY

Down:
1. CUTS
3. DIAGNOSIS
4. BRUSEE
5. WEAK
7. TOOL
8. VARICOSE

4 — INTERNAL ORGANS

Across:
1. ILEOCECAL
5. PANCREAS
7. LIVER
9. SOLARPLEXUS
12. THROAT
13. DIAPHRAGM

Down:
2. APPENDIX
3. GALLBLADDER
4. KIDNEY
6. HEART
8. BLADDER
10. LUNGS
11. URETER

7 — BONES & JOINTS

Across:
3. JAW
5. SHOULDERJOINT
8. COCCYX
9. LUMBAR
12. KNEE
13. CERVICAL

Down:
1. HIP / HAND
2. FOOT
4. WRIST
6. RIBS
7. THORACIC
10. ANKLE
11. SKULL
Down:
SACRUM

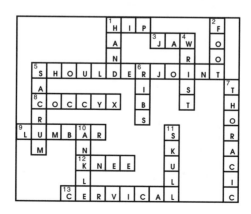

PUZZLE SOLUTIONS

CAUTIONS

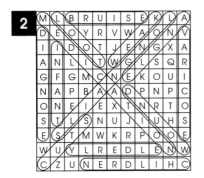
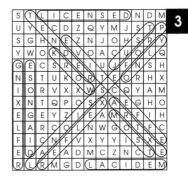

INTERNAL ORGANS

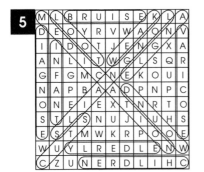
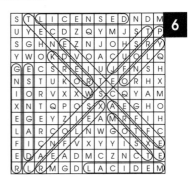

BONES & JOINTS

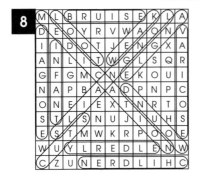
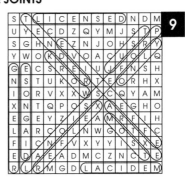

10

REFLEXOLOGY

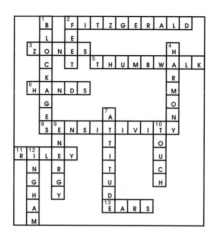

WELL BEING

11

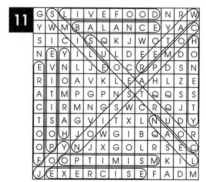

DIS - EASE

12

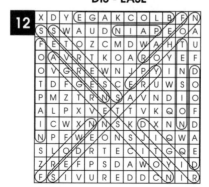

F.Y.I.

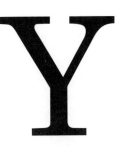

FOR YOUR INFORMATION

Presentation to the 2nd China Reflexology Symposium
October 16th, 1994-Beijing, China

INTRODUCTION

One of the most neglected aspects of the healing arts is the administration of health care to infants. Caring for infants poses particular problems since they are not able to communicate in language about their health status. The usual response to discomforts is crying which can often lead to additional internal stresses for the infant, including the effects of disturbed energy transmitted by a parent who feels helpless with the situation. Infants are receptive to natural healing, with relaxation for the infant being a very powerful way to address the source of their discomforts. Adults usually support the discomforts of

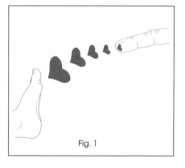

Fig. 1

an infant by holding and stroking actions on the head and body. The feet might only be touched casually, but they have unique pathways for relaxation which should be used. This discussion proposes a soothing and non-invasive technique of reflex action through the feet. The technique can be used exclusively for the infant's health, or as a support technique to break through the atmosphere of stress between a parent and infant where the health status might be interdependent.

ASSUMPTIONS

• Infants draw in less energy from the earth until the time they walk,

• Conventional reflexology has limitations for infants because of tender spots,

• The stress level of an adult may be linked to the stress level or discomfort of their infant,

• Infants are highly receptive to the energy transmitted through the emotions and thoughts of an adult,

• The potential for energetic balancing is greatly enhanced by inducing deep relaxation and normalizing sleep.

TECHNIQUE - Light Touch Reflex Action - (LTRA)

The technique described in this paper is based on The Metamorphic Technique of reflexology, as pioneered by Robert St. John of England. St. John's technique specifies foot, hand and head reflexing which concentrates on spinal and spinal cord reflexes to balance central nervous system pathways (fig. 2). For the purposes of reflexing for infants, I've found that sufficient stimulus or sedation is available through the foot reflexes alone. I've also been

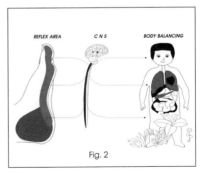

REFLEX AREA   C N S   BODY BALANCING

Fig. 2

guided by my own child to modify a regular light touch thumb walk technique into a circular touch

...continued next page

technique which can be used on the foot, or on top of the socks or infant clothing that covers the feet.

Cautions - As with any touch modality, the person administering the reflex action should pay attention to, and respect the energies and subtleties of inter-acting with family bonds. This technique may prove to be difficult or impossible if the family bonds are dys-functional, or the prevailing cultural or religious beliefs question the interactions of a foreign 'energy'. In such situations a member of the family should be instructed on how to reflex for the child. While an infant is awake, the feet and legs are very often in motion, and when LTRA is attempted, the infant motion might increase. It is a normal reaction of the adult 'giver' to think that the infant is rejecting the energetic stimulus at first, and for the adult to feel rejected by the infant. This should not be the case. The foot of the infant is rich in nerve endings, and the LTRA is something new for the infant to consciously assimilate.

Attitude - The touch itself is very light on the foot, very subtle, like the action of caressing a flower petal. The attitude is one of love and compassion. It is not necessary to focus on symptoms, but rather to let the fullness of the 'giver's' compassion focus onto the medial aspect of the foot. The 'giver' should attempt to clear or center their own energies as best possible before entering the energetic boundaries of the in-fant. When the energetic link is established through the action of the fingers on the foot, there is often a visible response from the infant. It could be stimulative or sedative depending on the circumstances and level of internal or external energetic stress present.

LIGHT TOUCH REFLEX ACTION

Technique - The thumb or fingers are used to make very slow circular movements along the medial aspect of the foot, letting the thumb or fingers travel up and down without any particular focus.

•The most effective **areas** to reflex are:

1. The spinal reflex from toe to heel.

2. The pelvic reflex area under and around the medial ankle bone. (see fig. 3).

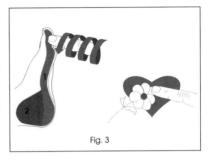
Fig. 3

•The reflex **action** on the foot is:

1. Light on the skin surface, and
2. A circular motion with a finger, fingers or a thumb; a little larger in diameter than the size of the finger or thumb itself. The speed of rotation should be slow and smooth, as if to transmit the love and compassion through the touch of the 'giver' (see fig. 1 & 3).

Reactions - Reactions to a session of reflexing generally fall into two categories.
1. Sedation.
2. Stimulation.

For infants, as with adults, there can be energetic rebalancing. For an infant this can be most evident in changes in sleep patterns, especially after the first session of reflexing. The infant might sleep more or less, or wake up more times than usual, especially with the first session.

...continued next page

Other reactions may include any of the accepted reactions encountered for adult reflexing, including:

1. Release of toxins from the body,
2. A period of increased or decreased physical activity, and,
3. A period where the ailment or discomfort gets a little more acute before getting better.

GUIDELINES FOR LTRA FOR INFANTS

1.   A hand puppet or toy may be necessary to distract the infant while one foot is being reflexed. This is particularly useful for a first session when the energies of 'giver' and 'receiver' are new to each other. The distraction can be introduced first, and then the reflex action is started after the infant has accepted the 'giver' into its energy boundaries.

2.   When the foot of an infant is approached for the first time, the initial reactions of the infant might be quite energetic, with crying or increased crying if the infant was already crying. The reflex action should be maintained by following the foot with the touch contact as best as possible.

3.   If the infant pulls one foot away, work on the other one, then come back to the first one. Follow the foot with your fingers if there is much motion from the infant. Sometimes the infant might show strong signs of only wanting one of the feet reflexed. This appears to be a possible and normal reaction, and the 'giver' should honor the unconscious mechanisms that are at work for the infant.

4. Reflex for as much time as the infant seems to want, or the 'giver' feels like doing. Length of time can be for 5-15 minutes, or until a visible shift in energy is noticed.

5. An infant spends much time in sleep. Reflexing at this time can be very effective and advantageous since the infant's conscious mechanisms are not involved. LTRA is so non-invasive and relaxing that sleep is rarely interrupted by the reflex action. But if the sleep is interrupted, it should resume quickly. It should be noted that the infant's body might twitch during LTRA, indicating nerve release.

6. The technique seems to be most effective when the 'giver' remains clear of willful intent to address specific symptoms.

CONCLUSION

Infants are vulnerable to sickness and disease, but they can also be vulnerable to healing remedies. The widespread use of antibiotics has recently been exposed (in the U.S.) to be a matter of high concern. A natural touch therapy such as LTRA can be a tremendous assist for balancing the body functions of infants, and boosting natural immune functions. LTRA can be a further help in addressing stresses within family bonds where a parent's ailments might be linked to the health of the infant.

What is a reflex tool? Basically, it's anything you use to **apply pressure** to reflexes other than your own touch. The term 'reflex tool' is new, but actually the concept has been around for a long time. Prayer beads and rosary beads are the most notable, providing relaxation and comfort for many people around the world. Just ask someone who uses them if they wish to part with them! These beads are usually held in the hand and manipulated or counted with an action which applies pressure between the index finger and thumb. Why are they a comfort and source of relaxation? Well, the pituitary gland reflex happens to be in the fleshy part of the thumb, as it is for the great toe on the foot. The beads apply pressure in this area when they're manipulated. Remember that the pituitary reflex is a powerful reflex for stress reduction... so it's really no wonder that people become so very attached to them.

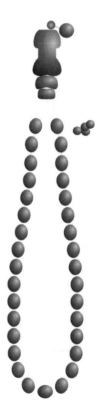

You already have many things around you that can **substitute** for your touch if needed. It could be a rounded wooden object, a golf ball. Remember the ball, stair treads and stones at the beginning of the book? The list could be endless.

There are many **commercially** available items as well: foot rollers, rubber-spiked balls, mini-massagers, electric vibrating pads, foot baths. Specialty stores, TV advertisements, massage suppliers, or self-care catalogs are good sources for these items.

These tools can be extremely useful, but remember that the **human touch** energy is missing when they're used. However, a persons' hand or thumb may be too weak for effective reflexing, or long nails may get in the way, or you need to reach a spot without doing a contortion act to position a thumb or finger on the reflex. In such cases a tool can be quite useful.

These tools, however, should be thought of as **self-care tools.** By using a tool on another person you might over stimulate a reflex since you're not really **in touch** with it... so to speak. You loose the **feedback** through your touch about the tender spots! Just think about how you react to a hand shake. Most handshakes are comfortable. Then there's the vice-grip, and then there's the old hidden buzzer trick device that shocks the living daylights out of you because you had no idea what was coming.

General guidelines for **working the feet** with tools is outlined on the next pages. Implements come in many shapes, sizes and materials. Some are designed for working one foot at a time; other types may work both feet together. It's largely a matter of personal feel. Each design can be quite a different experience on your feet... and on your body!

...continued next page

Once you fit this activity into your life, however, you just might make it a **habit like brushing your teeth...** and start a collection of rollers since each design may reflex quite differently. A roller that feels good for a teenager might not be comfortable for a senior citizen. A roller that works well for a person in normal health might not feel appropriate for someone with a chronic ailment. Above all, remember that everybody has different sensitivities, so the type of contact that a tool makes with a foot may feel different for each person... just like the human touch!

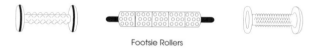

Footsie Rollers

Electric stimulating devices come in all kinds of variations. There are 'body tools' that may be adapted for use on the feet, and others that are specific for the feet. All of them usually have speed or vibration settings, and some even have heat!

Two main variations on electric devices are:

1. Hand-held devices that have vibrating knobs.
2. Floor units that have stimulating pads or rolling balls under a soft cover.

   a. The types that have pads make a general stimulus to the reflexes.

   b. The ones with rollers work the reflexes much deeper.

The guidelines and cautions for footsie rollers also apply to electric devices, along with the manufacturers' directions or recommendations.

FOOTSIE ROLLERS

1   **Sit in a chair to roll the feet.**

NEVER put your **FULL WEIGHT** on a roller or electrical device! Don't stand on it or leave it around to be tripped over! **If you choose** to apply pressure while standing, use the back of a chair or something solid to hold on to. This will help minimize a full weight transfer to the roller.

2   **Roll the feet**

The most effective rolling is done barefoot, but if your feet feel overly sensitive, you might try with a pair of thick socks. Place a roller on the floor and start by rolling the **sole** of a foot back and forth from toe to heel. Take note of where the most tender spots are. Rolling one foot at a time allows you to concentrate on the reflexes. After spending extra time on tender spots, roll the broader areas to smooth out the stimulus. The toes and heel are difficult to roll, but you can apply **pressure** to these reflexes in the following manner:
• for the **toes,** grasp the roller with your toes and push into the roller with your heel flat on the ground,
• for the **heel,** roll slowly back and forth in small areas.

3   **Roll on 3 sides**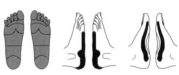

You'll probably roll the soles of the feet the most. It feels the best! Nevertheless don't neglect the sides of the feet since they hold reflexes to 75 percent of the bones of the body among other reflexes! Remember the **rule of thumb** for reflexing: start off lighter and gradually work with more pressure, adjusting both the pressure and the time for your own personal comfort.

A **general guide** for rolling (mechanical or electrical), is :
• to reflex more vigorously in the morning or during the day
   - *for stimulus* - 2-5 minutes
• to reflex more gently in the evening
   - *for relaxation* - 5-15 minutes or more.

If reflexology can be thought of as any one thing, it's an **exploration**, truly an adventure allowing us to communicate with our own body. Reflexes have incredible potentials for communicating, just like telephone or computer keyboards. And like for the keyboards, you must apply your touch, to make the connection!

Actually we can think of ourselves as bundles of reflex pathways that are constantly reacting to events and information surrounding us, which then gets translated into our inner environment... our body and mind.

Just as no two people are the same in character and sensitivities, so there are no firm rules for reflexing... but there are many valid guidelines. The time you invest will develop your own hidden talents for using your touch in a consistent and beneficial manner. Be patient, and be **comfortable** with your reflexing. Be humble, and be compassionate with your touch. We all have this **gift** within us, it's just a matter of using it! Whether it be for a birth, or a passing on from this earth, there's an appropriate and effective manner to reflex for all, and rewards to cherish whatever the age:

• for the very young who can't yet communicate, it's a relaxing connection to healing energies,

• for children, reflexing is a way of investing in their health, through their feet... along with the positive attitudes concerning the touch,

• for teenagers, the adventure can be truly empowering, a way of balancing the body and mind at a time when there are so many questions about life,

• for adults, most of whom bear the heaviest responsibilities, health-care is not only an issue, but also an economic burden of its own,

• for those of the golden age, the touch work brings forth caring attitudes which are so often lacking to our youth-oriented, fast-paced world that often leaves them so very far behind.

I've spent the past eleven years exploring the powerful benefits associated with reflexology. I've come into contact with people of all walks of life, in many countries, all of whom have cherished the modality for it's safe and effec-tive action on the body and mind. Being a professional re-flexologist and instructor of re-flexology, I'm often asked what the mo-dality is good for, what it can really do, what specific ben-

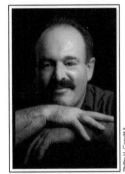

efits can be derived. I prefer to make no claims, choosing instead to explain how the body has a chance to balance its own energies when given a chance. And it needs this chance on a daily basis! We're constantly attempting to 'recover' from something. Whether it be a head or tooth ache, back pain, tennis elbow, tired eyes or a stuffed up nose, a digestive disturbance, the common cold, and of course the proverbial pain in the neck (our own, or coming from something or someone else as a source of aggravation)...

... health issues are always an issue!

...continued next page

Another question I'm often asked is how reflexology works, what's the scientific explanation? Unfortunately, there's no single consensus or theory concerning this. All of the theories have validities, but then, do we need to know how an aspirin works in order to benefit from it. One brand (label) of aspirin usually works better for a person than another brand, right? The aspirin analogy is useful for reflexology. You don't have to understand its mechanisms for it to work, but the kind of touch you use might very well **label** the kind of reflexing that's best for you.

Still another question concerns the touch itself. We've all heard the expression 'healing hands". Actually, everyone's touch is a bit different, since our thought patterns have a lot to do with it. Since reflexology depends so much on human touch, it pays to let your touch be **human**.

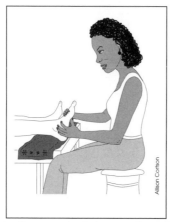

Energy, whether in the form of touch or the thoughts behind the touch, knows no boundaries. It rises above color, creed, age or status in life. Whether for yourself or for another person, reflexing brings forth a wonderful sense of empowerment... the ability to **care** for health with your own simple touch. Explore this gift, use it with vitality... the rewards will amaze you!

Hopefully you'll have the motivation and courage to put reflexing to work for you , to make it an adventurous part of your life, as consistent as brushing your teeth perhaps, but far more exciting. Don't let **preconceived** ideas about the feet get in your way either. They carry you through life and reflect every stimulus that enters you. Honor them! And don't worry about your touch or about the maps. Reflexing is forgiving, and it's honest. Remember that those tender spots are giving you feedback. Listen to them... be in touch with them... let them **communicate** with you.

The future is bright for reflexology, both as a self-help health care technique, and as a profession unto itself. It's literally bursting forth around the globe, coming forward from it's ancient roots... expanding into the field of **complementary** health care at a rapid rate, and opening up new frontiers for balancing the functions of the body and mind.

Reflexology has an inherent **simplicity** which is often misleading. Simple touch. Simple actions. Simple beneficial reactions. But rising above this simplicity is the fact that it leads to a balancing of energies, and perhaps even to a place of relaxation that can be a sanctuary for our **souls**, a place to commune with the greatest healer of all...

the power of the **universe**.

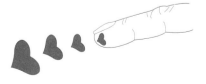

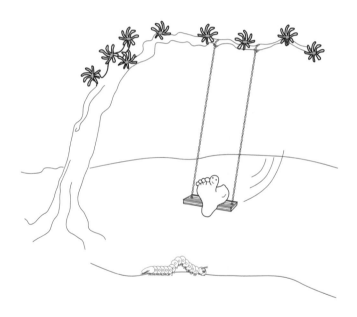

Now that you've started getting in touch with your feet... honor this **gift** that lies within your body by fitting it into your life in a comfortable manner.

Remember that the most effective reflexing is done by working the **broader areas.** You've learned how to navigate ... so smooth sailing and keep me handy to refer to.

I can be a friend for life!

Until later...

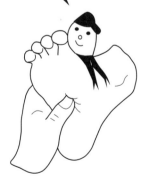

Z

INDEXES

REFLEXOLOGY ASSOCIATIONS

Reflexology is widely practised around the world. The following list may be helpful to you if you are seeking more information about reflexology including certification courses, basic hands-on workshops, association newsletters, referals to certified practitioners, or speaking forums. Please note that a self addressed stamped envelope might expedite your requests.

STATE LEVEL

Reflexology Association of California (RAC) P.O. Box 641156 Los Angeles, CA 90064	**CALIFORNIA**
Foot Reflexology Awareness Association (FRAA) P.O. Box 7622 Mission Hills, CA91346	
Associated Reflexologists of Colorado (ACR) P.O. Box 471812 Aurora, CO 80047	**COLORADO**
Iowa Association of Reflexologists (IAR) 1315 Hammond Ave. Waterloo, IA 50702	**IOWA**
Maine Council of Reflexologists (MCR) P.O. Box 969 Jefferson, ME 04348	**MAINE**
Missouri State Reflexology Association (MSRA) 12817 East 47th, 17 Grove Independence, MO 64055	**MISSOURI**
Nevada Reflexology Organization (NRO) 41Walhaven Court Las Vegas, NV 89103	**NEVADA**
North Dakota Reflexology Association (NDRA) P.O. Box 7 Edinburg, ND 58227	**NORTH DAKOTA**
Ohio Association of Reflexologists (OAR) P.O. Box 428725 Cincinnati, OH 45242	**OHIO**
Pennsylvania Reflexology Association (PRA) 1900 Emerson Street Philadelphia, PA 18951	**PENNSYLVANIA**
Reflexology Organization of Wisconsin (ROW) 904 Gail Place Fort Atkinson, WI 53538	**WISCONSIN**

NATIONAL LEVEL

Reflexology Association of America P. O. Box 162752 Sacramento, CA 95820	**U. S. A.**
American Reflexology Certification Board P. O. Box 620607 Littleton, CO 80162	**U. S. A.**

WORLDWIDE

Reflexology Association of Australia **AUSTRALIA**
P.O. Box 1032
Bondi Junction NSW 2022

Reflexology Association of Canada **CANADA**
11 Glen Cameron Road #4
Thornhill, Ontario L3T 4N3

China Reflexology Association **CHINA**
P.O. Box 2002
Beijing 100026

Zoneterapeutforeningen FDZ **DENMARK**
Chr. Winterhersvej 13
6000 Kolding

British Association of Reflexologists **ENGLAND**
Sillwood Mansions #6
Brighton BN1 2LH

Metamorphic Association
67 Ritherdon Road
London, S.W., 17-8QE

New Zealand Reflexology Association **NEW ZEALAND**
P.O. Box 31- 084
Milford, Aukland 9

Scottish Institute of Reflexology **SCOTLAND**
57 A Longhill Ave.
Ayr, KA7 4DY

South African Reflexology Association **SOUTH AFRICA**
P.O. Box 201858
Durban North 4016

Swiss Reflexology Association **SWITZERLAND**
Renan, CH 2616

Rwo-Shur Health Institute International **TAIWAN**
P.O. Box 826
Taipei, R. O. C.

International Council of Reflexologists (ICR) **U. S. A.**
P.O. Box 621963
Littleton, CO 80162

Abut, M. Fuat, Op. Dr. *Kulak Akupunkturu- Aurikulotherapie.* Istanbul, Turkey. Matbaa Teknisyenleri Basimevi, 1987.

Bayly, Doreen, E. *Reflexology Today-The Stimulation of The Body's Healing Forces Through Foot Massage.* Rochester, Vermont. Healing Arts Press, 1988.

Bear, Soaring. *Dental Self Help.* Just Deserts, Arizon. The Mother Duck Press, 1983.

Byers, Dwight C. *Better Health With Foot Reflexology-The Original Ingham Method ™.* St. Petersburg, Florida. Ingham Publishing, 1983.

Carter, Mildred. *Body Reflexology, Healing at Your Fingertips.* West Nyack, N.Y. Parker Publishing Co. 1983.

Carter, Mildred. *Hand Reflexology, Key to Perfect Health.* West Nyack, N.Y. Parker Publishing Co., 1975.

China Reconstruct Press. *Practical Ways to Good Health Through Chinese Traditional Medicine.* Beijing, China. Foreign Language Printing House, 1989.

Davidson, John. *Subtle Energy.* Saffron Walden, England. The C.W. Daniel Co. Ltd., 1987.

Davis, Albert R. & Rawls, Walter C. Jr. *The Rainbow In Your Hands.* Kansas City, Missouri. Acres Publishing, 1992.

Dobbs, B., Paratte, D., Poletti, R. *Réflexologie.* Geneva, Switzerland. Editions Sophia, 1987.

Dougans, Inge with Ellis, Suzane. *Reflexology-Foot Massage for Total Health.* Rockport, Massachusetts. Element, Inc., 1991.

Dougans, Inge with Ellis, Suzane. *The Art of Reflexology.* Rockport, Massachusetts. Element, Inc., 1992.

Eastman, Yvette. *Touchpoint Reflexology - The First Steps.* Campbell River, Canada. Ptarmigan Press, 1991.

Eisenberg, David, M.D., with Wright, Thomas L., *Encounters With Qi.* New York, N.Y., Penguin Books, 1985.

Fitztgerald, W. H., M.D. *Zone Therapy.* Mokelumne Hill, California. Health Research, 1917.

Gagnieux, Pierre L. *Réflexologie, Tome 1 Théorique-Les pieds et le Corps Mis à Nus.* Laval, Canada. Guy Saint-Jean Editeur Inc, 1991.

Gagnieux, Pierre L. *Réflexologie, Tome 2 Pratique.* Laval, Canada. Guy Saint-Jean Editeur Inc, 1991.

Goosmann-Legger, Astrid I. *Zone Therapy Using Foot Massage.* Saffron Walden, England. The C.W. Daniel Co., 1992

Grinberg, Avi. *Foot Analysis-The foot Path to Self-Discovery.* York Beach, Maine. Samuel Weiser, Inc., 1993.

Grinberg, Avi. *Holistic Reflexology.* Wellingborough, England. Thorsons Publishers, 1989.

Ingham, Eunice D. *Stories the Feet Can Tell Thru Reflexology/Stories the Feet Have Told Thru Reflexology.* St. Petersburg, Florida. Ingham Publishing, 1984.

Issel, Christine. *Reflexology: Art, Science & History.* Sacramento, California. New Frontier Publishing, 1990

Krasensky, Jean-Pierre. *Massage Réflexe des Pieds.* St-Jean-de-Braye, France. Editions Dangles, 1987.

Kunz, Kevin & Kunz, Barbara. *Hand and Foot Reflexology-A Self-Help Guide.* New York, N.Y. Simon & Schuster, 1984.

Kunz, Kevin & Kunz, Barbara. *The Complete Guide to Foot Reflexology.* New York, N.Y. Prentiss Hall Press, 1987.

Lust, Benedict, M.D. *Zone Therapy-Relieving Pain and Sickness by Nerve Pressure.* New York, N.Y. Benedict Lust Publications, 1980.

Manning, Clark A. & Vanrenen, Louis J. *Bioenergetic Medicines East and West.* Berkeley, California. North Atlantic Books, 1988.

Marquardt, Hanne. *Reflex Zone Therapy Of The Feet-A Textbook For Therapists.* Rochester, Vermaont. Healing Art Press, 1984.

Norman, Laura, with Cowan, Thomas. *Feet First-A Guide To Foot Reflexology.* New York, New York. Simon & Schuster Inc., 1988.

Oleson, Terry, PhD. & Flocco, William. *Randomized controlled study of premenstrual symptoms treated with ear, hand and foot reflexology.* Obstet & Gynecol, 1993 Dec 82:906-11

Riley, Joe S. Dr., Daglish, W.E. *Zone Reflex.* Mokelumne Hill, California. Health Research, 1961.

Rogers, Sandi. *Professional Reflexology for Everyone.* Victoria, Australia. The Victorian School of Reflexology & Herbal Studies, 1992.

Segal, Maybelle. *Reflexology.* North Hollywood, California. Melvin Powers Wishire Book Co., 1976.

Saint-Pierre,Gaston&Shapiro,Debbie. *The Metamorphic Technique-Principles and Practice.* Shaftesbury, England. Element Books, 1982.

Turgeon, Madeleine. *Découvrons La Réflexologie-Technique d'Acupuncture Sans Aiguilles.* Boucherville, Canada. Editions de Mortagne, 1986.

Turgeon, Madeleine. *Energie it Réflexologie-La Polarité à Votre Portée.* Boucherville, Canada. Editions de Mortagne, 1985.

Turgeon, Madeleine. *La Réflexologie Du Cerveau-Pour Auditifs et Visuels.* Boucherville, Canada. Editions de Mortagne, 1988.

Volf, Nadia, Dr. *Vos Mains Sont Votre Premier Médecin.* Maxéville, France. Editions Fixot, 1994.

Wagner, Franz Ph.D., Reflex Zone Massage-Handbook of Therapy and Self-Help. Wellingborough, England. Thorsons Publishing, 1987

Wills, Pauline. *The Reflexology & Colour Therapy Workbook.* Rockport, Massachusetts. Element, Inc, 1992.

INDEX